A TREATISE OF
MELANCHOLIE

PUBLICATION NO. 50 OF
THE FACSIMILE TEXT SOCIETY

A TREATISE OF MELANCHOLIE

By T. BRIGHT

Reproduced from the 1586 edition printed by Thomas Vautrollier, with an introduction by HARDIN CRAIG

Published for
THE FACSIMILE TEXT SOCIETY
By COLUMBIA UNIVERSITY PRESS
NEW YORK : M·CM·XL

COPYRIGHT, 1940
COLUMBIA UNIVERSITY PRESS, NEW YORK

Foreign agents: OXFORD UNIVERSITY PRESS, Humphrey Milford, Amen House, London, E.C. 4, England, AND B. I. Building, Nicol Road, Bombay, India, MARUZEN COMPANY, LTD., 6 Nihonbashi, Tori-Nichome, Tokyo, Japan

MANUFACTURED IN THE UNITED STATES OF AMERICA

INTRODUCTION

THE WORD "melancholy" meant to the Elizabethans, as to us also, not only settled depression, sadness, downcast and dispirited dejection, distress, misery, and hysteria, but also disease itself, not merely the symptoms of disease. It was a disordered condition of the body believed to be due to excess of black bile. This was natural melancholy. There was also unnatural melancholy, arising from a disordered physical condition of black bile itself, of choler, of blood, or even of phlegm, though a disordered condition of phlegm as a cause of unnatural melancholy was in dispute. The earlier pages of Bright's *Treatise of Melancholie* will make this clear.

Gloominess was the primary symptom of the disease of melancholy, but irascibility, sullenness, despondency, hypochrondria, morbidity, frenzy, and madness were also symptoms. These symptoms were and are very general in human life. Galen and his followers in medical science made the not unusual mistake of seeking one cause for one set of symptoms which arise from various causes, just as at the present time men seek cures for headaches and colds. The study of melancholy thus became a sort of baffled exploration of the superficies of the vaguer sorts of human suffering. The erroneous hypothesis of the four humors and four qualities might do well enough for the delineation of general classes of passions and sufferings; but like all false hypotheses it required, as soon as it was specifically applied, to be patched and adjusted. Consequently it grew complex in nature and covered an area at once too vague and too extensive.

Our ancestors knew little enough

about diet, and there was much error mixed with their knowledge. We know that their food was inadequate in variety and often unwholesome. We know that they ate too much—as we do. Their livers and kidneys must habitually have undergone great injury, and in consequence all sorts of distressing things must have happened to their hearts, their brains, and their nervous systems. In his *Treatise* Bright pays much attention to diet, and in that respect he is on the right track and is in some measure original. The men of Bright's time were unhygienically clothed and badly housed. Their medication was almost worse than useless. They grouped many ailments together and said, "I am melancholy," which was equivalent to saying, "I am alive and I am not happy." The only course they knew was to analyze that state. They learned that melancholy people were not stupid, except with a certain sort of stupidity, that they were likely to be brave, witty, and thoughtful, and that they were liable to delusions and to frenzy and madness. They had no way of particularizing except to observe, to study, and to expand. This kind of study was Bright's task, and he did it well.

The subject of melancholy was an old one. A competently trained physician could talk about the subject and write treatises about it merely on the basis of what he had learned in the university, his reading, and his experience as a physician. The fact that Burton cites such multitudes of authorities in his *Anatomy of Melancholy* makes the writing of a treatise on melancholy seem an affair of special learning; but it was not so. Many physicians can and do write whole books on various aspects of medicine, particularly of popular medicine, without finding it necessary to quote authorities. They merely draw on the great reservoir of medical knowledge which, as trained physicians, they have learned from various sources. Of their particular subjects they give their own versions; and this is what Timothy Bright did. He refers a number of times to Galen, whose *De melancholia, sive atrae bilis morbo* was the basis of the subject of melancholy. Bright's *Treatise* and, no doubt, all treatises on melancholy derive their form from Galen—definitions, symptoms, kinds, causes, and cures. Bright doubtless knew other books on melancholy. He refers casually to Aëtius on page 215. He probably knew the Hippocratic works, *De humoribus* and *De vulneribus capitis*, Constantinus Africanus, *De melancholia*, and the works of Levinus Lemnius, whose *Touchstone of Complexions* appeared in English translation in 1576. How many other books in Burton's great list Bright knew there is no way of telling. Caelius Aurelianus, Melanelius, Prosper Calenus, Rodericus à Fonseca, Thomas Erastus, Jason Pratensis, and half a dozen others lay, no doubt, in his way. It would be interesting to know if Bright was acquainted with Melanchthon, Vives, Cardan, and Paracelsus.

Timothy Bright wrote as an authority on a well-known subject, and as such he took his place with his contemporaries. And yet in saying this, one has not finished with Galen. From the earliest times there had been a difference of opinion as to the relation of the soul and the body to the sufferings due to melancholy. Burton (Pt. I, sec. 2, memb. 5, subsec. 1) states the issue as follows:

For as the distraction of the mind, amongst other outward causes and perturbations, alters the temperature of the body, so the distraction and distemper of the body will cause a distemperature of the soul: & 'tis hard to

INTRODUCTION

decide which of these two do most harm to the other. *Plato, Cyprian,* & some others . . . lay the greatest fault upon the soul, excusing the body; others again, accusing the body, excuse the soul, as a principal agent. Their reasons are, because *the manners do follow the temperature of the body,* as Galen proves in his book of that subject, *Prosper Calenius, de Atra Bile, Jason Pratensis, c. de Mania, Lemnius, l.* 4, *c.* 16, and many others. And that which *Gualter* hath commented, *hom.* 10 *in epist. Johannis,* is most true; concupiscence and original sin, inclinations, and bad humours, are radical in every one of us, causing these perturbations, affections, and several distempers, offering many times violence unto the soul.

The Platonic position was that the soul is untouchable by physical causes and, if it does its duty through the will as the agent of an enlightened reason, may and should protect the body from suffering. It might thus be said that in melancholy the soul has by neglect injured the body. This point of view is implicit in such works as Cardan's *De consolatione*. The Galenic position is the more familiar one. According to it the ills of the body affect the well-being of the soul, drive it into misery and madness, so that it may be said that the body injures the soul. All treatises on melancholy as a disease are more or less Galenic.

Under the impulse of an age turning more and more to science there was in all branches of medicine a great wave of Galenism in the late sixteenth and the early seventeenth centuries. From it came Vesalius, Burton, and Harvey. Bright also belongs to this wave of Galenism, although it was perhaps his reservations against Galenism that caused him to write at all. Bright was a student of divinity as well as medicine. He gave up the cure of bodies for the cure of souls, and on June 8, 1591, we find him

INTRODUCTION xiii

installed as rector of Methley, in Yorkshire.[1] Although he believed with Galen that melancholy is a disease and therefore subject to medical treatment, he was unwilling completely to accept Galenic materialism. He wished to provide a ground for the operation of his theology and therefore wrote his *Treatise of Melancholie* to show that, although Galenic therapeutics of melancholy was excellent and applicable, it might not be made to include contrition and those stings of conscience which God himself chooses to inflict on the sinner. Beyond this reservation there is nothing to withhold Bright from the society of writers on melancholy who became more and more numerous until Burton's time. Many of Burton's favorite authors, such as Franciscus Hildesheim, Hercules de

[1] For the facts of Bright's life see William J. Carlton, *Timothe Bright Doctor of Phisicke*, London, 1911.

Saxonia, Felix Plater, André du Laurens, Montaltus, Heurnius, Huarte Navarro, Thomas Wright, and Bishop John Abernethy, had not yet written.[2]

It must also be understood that the subject of melancholy took on new aspects during this period of intense exploitation. Medical interest continued. Huarte and others applied the doctrine of the humors to the choice of professions. Ben Jonson and others applied it to the presentation of character in drama [3] Many writers used the doctrine of the humors and faculty psychology (not then so-called) in the expression and delineation of passion. Bright's *Treatise* is an early simple handbook—

[2] For an account of Burton's sources see Paul Jordan-Smith, *Bibliographia Burtoniana*. Stanford University, 1931.

[3] See Percy Simpson's introduction to *Everyman in His Humour* and to *Everyman out of His Humour* in *Ben Jonson*, ed. by Herford and Simpson, Vol. I.

at the opposite extreme from Burton's *Anatomy*. It will serve to show the principles from which the literature of melancholy developed. With Bright melancholy was not a mood; it was a disease. It had become a mood in the tragedies of Shakespeare and the comedies of Jonson, in contemporary writings, and to a considerable extent in the work of Burton; although to Burton melancholy was also a disease. Nashe knew the subject well, and perhaps he, Marston, Donne, Breton, and Burton (by his own confession) furnish us examples of melancholic careers. We cannot rob these men of a genuine feeling that life was futile, for gloom hung heavily over the period. Shakespeare mocks at melancholy in his early plays, but not in *Hamlet*, *King Lear*, and *Timon of Athens*.[4]

[4] See "An Essay on Elizabethan Melancholy," in G. B. Harrison's edition of Nicholas Breton's *Melancholike Humours*, London, 1929.

Shakespeare may have known Bright's *Treatise of Melancholie*. It was available, simple, and authoritative. The stock of Thomas Vautrollier passed into the hands of Richard Field, Shakespeare's fellow townsman and the publisher of *Venus and Adonis* and *The Rape of Lucrece*. The accurate description of melancholic symptoms in *Hamlet* and other plays reminds one of Bright. In *Hamlet* and in the sonnets there are a number of fairly close verbal echoes.[5] But the question is not easily solved, since a good deal of the phraseology is current medical language and since the knowledge which Shakespeare possessed was also available in a number of other works, such as those of Lemnius, Boaistuau, La Primaudaye, Huarte Navarro, and various others. Neverthe-

---

[5] See Mary Isabelle O'Sullivan, "Hamlet and Dr. Timothy Bright," *Publications of the Modern Language Association of America*, XLI, 667-79.

less the case for Shakespeare's having known Bright is good.

A Treatise of Melancholie came out in three editions:

1. A TREATISE OF MELAN-CHOLIE. LONDON, *by Thomas Vautrollier*, 1586.

COLLATION BY SIGNATURES: *, 8 leaves; **, 4 leaves; A, B, C, D, E, F, G, H, I, K, L, M, N, O, P, Q, R, S, each 8 leaves; total 156 numbered leaves. Leaf [**iij] has no signature mark.

COLLATION BY PAGINATION: [title], |A| TREATISE OF | MELANCHOLIE. | CONTAINING THE CAVSES | thereof, & reasons of the strange effects it worketh | in our minds and bodies: with the phisicke cure, and | spirituall consolation for such as haue thereto ad- | ioyned an afflicted conscience. | *The difference betwixt it, and melancholie with diuerse* | *philosophical discourses touching actions, and af-* | *fections of soule, spirit, and body: the par-* | *ticulars whereof are to be seene* | *before the booke.* | By T. Bright

Doctor of Phisicke. | [printer's device — McKerrow 164] | Imprinted at London by Thomas Vautrol- | lier, dwelling in the Black- | Friers. 1586. |, recto of [*]; — [blank], verso of [*]; — | [type-ornament head-piece] | TO THE RIGHT | VVOR-SHIPFVL M. | PETER OSBOVRNE, &c. | [signed] | *A louer of your vertue,* | T. Bright. |, recto of *ij to verso of [*v]; — | [type-ornament head-piece] | TO HIS MELAN- | cholicke friend: M. |, recto of [*vi] to recto of **; — [blank], verso of **; — | [type-ornament head-piece] | *THE CONTENTES OF* | *the booke according to the* | *Chapters.* |, recto of **ij to verso of **iiij; — [text, with heading], | [type-ornament head-piece] | A TREA-TISE | OF MELAN- | CHOLIE. |, pp. 1–284; — | FINIS. |, p. 284; — | *Faults escaped in the printing . . .* | p. [285]; — [blank], p. [286].

Page 25 is wrongly marked 35; 28 is 12; 102 is 82; 124 is 114; 138 is 158; 191 is 190; 222 is .22; 223 and 224 are repeated; 252 is wrongly numbered 250; 253 is 251;

255 is 125; 273 is 173; 280 is 266; 281 is 280.

Catchword on p. 144 is "hinder" instead of "the"; on p. 160, "large" (wrong) instead of "are"; on p. 224, "ding" (right) instead of "glorie"; and on p. 246 it is "Of" instead of "all."

CONDITION: Size of leaf, 5 9/16 x 3 13/16 inches; 14.2 x 9.7 centimetres. Bound in brown crushed levant, gilt back, sides, inside borders, and edges; by the Club Bindery, 1901.

The Hoe copy, with ex-libris; now in the Huntington Library. This copy has been reproduced in the following facsimile.

2. A TREATISE OF MELANCHOLY. LONDON, *by Iohn VVindet*, 1586.

COLLATION BY SIGNATURES: *, 8 leaves; A, B, C, D, E, F, G, H, I, K, L, M, N, O, P, Q, R, each 8 leaves; S, 2 leaves; total, 146 numbered leaves. Leaf [Biiij] is numbered Biii. Leaves [Mii], [Miii], and [Miiii] are numbered, respectively, M2, M3, and M4.

COLLATION BY PAGINATION: [title], | *A* TREATISE OF | *MELANCHOLY.* | Contayning the causes thereof, and | reasons of the straunge effects it worketh in our | *minds and bodies: with the Phisicke cure, and* | *spirituall consolation for such as haue* | *thereto adioyned afflicted* | *conscience.* | *The difference betwixt it, and melancholy, with di-* | *uerse philosophicall discourses touching actions, and* | *affections of soule, spirit and body: the particu-* | *lars whereof are to be seene before* | *the booke.* | By T. Bright Doctor of | Phisicke. | [printer's device] | Imprinted at London by | Iohn VVindet. | 1586. |, recto of [*]; [blank], verso of [*]; | TO THE RIGHT | WORSHIPFVL M. PE | TER OSBOVRNE. &c. | [signed] *A louer of your vertue*, T. Bright. |, recto of *ij to verso of *iij; | *TO HIS ME-* | lancholick friend M. |, recto of *iiij to recto of [*v]; | [blank], verso of [*v]; | [type-ornament headpiece] | THE CONTENTES OF | the booke according to the | Chapters. |, recto of [*vi] to recto of [*viij]; | [blank], verso of [*viij]; |

[text, with heading], | [type-ornament headpiece] | A TREATISE | OF MELAN- | CHOLIE. | , pp. 1– [276]; | FINIS. | , p. [276].

No irregularities in catchwords or pagination. Size of leaf: 5$\frac{5}{16}$ x 3$\frac{10}{16}$ inches; 13.5 x 9 centimetres. Bound in maroon russia. Gilt back, sides, inside borders & edges. Upper margins of pages 273–276 closely cropped, with loss of running titles and page numbers. Title page torn, no loss of lettering. Signature on foreleaf and date, 1837. Huntington Library copy used in this description and collation. Faults noted in Vautrollier edition are corrected in this.

3. An edition printed by William Stansby, 1613, follows the Windet edition in wording of title-page: "afflicted conscience" instead of "an afflicted conscience" as in Vautrollier edition. "Faults" are corrected. There are no other apparent differences in matter.

A Treatise of Melancholie thus went through two editions in the year of its publication and was sufficiently important to be reissued twenty-seven years later. Bright wrote a number of other medical works, including a commentary on the *Physica* of Scribonius. One of them, *A Treatise wherein is Declared the Sufficiencie of English Medicines*, was published twice in 1580 and again in 1615. He also contributed *Animadversiones de traduce* to the Ψυχολογία of Goclenius (1590). Burton treats Bright as an authority on melancholy with a good deal of respect. These facts seem to indicate that Bright enjoyed a considerable reputation as a scientist in his own day. His most lasting fame, however, comes from his invention of a system of shorthand writing. His well known *Characterie: an Arte of Shorte, Swifte, and Secrete Writing by Character* was published in 1588.

HARDIN CRAIG

Stanford University
Dec. 11, 1939

A TREATISE OF MELANCHOLIE

FACSIMILE

A TREATISE OF MELANCHOLIE.

CONTAINING THE CAVSES thereof, & reasons of the strange effects it worketh in our minds and bodies: with the phisicke cure, and spirituall consolation for such as haue thereto adioyned an afflicted conscience.

The difference betwixt it, and melancholie with diuerse philosophicall discourses touching actions, and affections of soule, spirit, and body: the particulars whereof are to be seene before the booke.

By T. Bright Doctor of Phisicke.

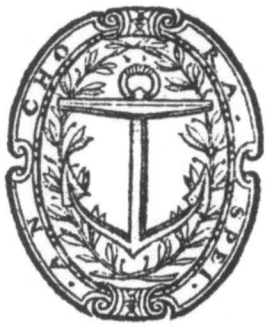

Imprinted at London by Thomas Vautrollier, dwelling in the Black-Friers. 1586.

TO THE RIGHT
VVORSHIPFVL M.
PETER OSBOVRNE, &c.

F all other pra-
ctise of phisick,
that parte most
cōmendeth the
excellēcy of the
noble facultie,
which not on-
ly releeueth the
bodily infirmity, but after a sort euen
also correcteth the infirmities of the
mind. For the instrument of reason,
the braine, being either not of well
tempered substance: or disordered in
his parts: all exercise of wisedome is
hindred: and where once vnderstanding lodged, wit, memorie, & quick

conceit, kept residence, and the excellencie of man appeareth aboue all other creatures: there vnconsiderate iudgement, simplicitie, & foolishnes make their seat, and as it were dispossessing reason, of her watch tower, subiecteth the nature of man vnto the annoyance of infinite calamities, that force vpõ vs in the course of this fraile life, & baseth it farre vnder the condition of brute beasts. The heart the seate of affection (and neither immoderate in temper, nor in figure or quantitie otherwise disposed then is expedient for good action) the seate of temperancie, of iustice, of fortitude and liberalitie, dayly practice of phisicke sheweth how much it is disposed and framed to mediocritie of affection wherin vertue consisteth, by such meanes as nature ministreth, & the phisitian hir great steward according to her will, dispenseth where need requireth: in so much that what
reason

DEDICATORIE.

reason bringeth to passe by perswasion and counsell, that medicine and other helpes of that kinde seeme to worke by instinct of nature. The dayly experience of phrensies, madnesse, lunasies, and melancholy cured by this heauenly gift of God, make manifest demonstration hereof. The notable fruit & successe of which art in that kinde, hath caused some to iudge more basely of the soule, then agreeth with pietie or nature, & haue accompted all maner affection thereof, to be subiect to the phisicians hãd, not considering herein any thing diuine, and aboue the ordinarie euents, and naturall course of thinges: but haue esteemed the vertues thẽ selues, yea religion, no other thing but as the body hath bẽ tempered, and on the other side, vice, prophanenesse, & neglect of religion and honestie, to haue bene nought else but a fault of humour. For correcting the iudge-

* iij

mēt of such as so greatly mistake the matter, and partly for the vse of many that may neede instruction and counsel, in the state of melancholy, & affection of braine and hart, & wold haue both to satisfie their owne doubts, and to answer the prophane obiections of others, I haue taken this paines to confute the absurde errour of the one, & to satisfie the reasonable and modest inquiry of the other that seek to be enformed. I haue layd open howe the bodie, and corporall things affect the soule, & how the body is affected of it againe: what the difference is betwixt natural melancholie, and that heauy hande of God vpon the afflicted conscience, tormented with remorse of sinne, & feare of his iudgement: with a Christian resolutiō according to my skill for such as faint vnder that heauie burthen. And that I might to the vttermost of my endeuor (as other businesse

finesse wold permit me) comfort thē
in that estate most comfortles, I haue
added mine aduise of phisicke helpe:
what diet, what medicine, and what
other remedie is meete for persons,
oppressed with melancholie feare, &
that kind of heauinesse of hart. I haue
enterlaced my treatise besides with
disputes of Philosophie that the learned sort of them, and such as are of
quicke conceit, & delited in discourse
of reason in naturall things, may find
to passe their time with, and knowe
the grounds and reasons of their passions, without which they might receaue more discomfort, and greater
cause of error. This I haue deliuered
in a simple phrase without any cost,
or port of words to a supposed frend
M. not ignorant of good letters, that
the discourse might be more familiar
then if it had caried other direction
it otherwise would be. Chaunge the
letter, and it is indifferent to whome

soeuer ſtandeth in need, or ſhal make vſe thereof. I write it in our mother tong that the benefit (how ſmall ſoeuer it be) might be more common, & as the practiſe of all auncient philoſophers hath ben to write in their owne language their precepts, whether concerning nature, or touching maners of life, to the end their countrey men might reape the benefite with more eaſe, and ſeeke rather for ſound iudgement of vnderſtanding, then for vaine oſtentation of ſtrange tongs: which is alſo after a ſort followed in tranſlations: ſo I tooke it meeteſt to impart theſe fewe poyntes of philoſophie, & phiſicke in Engliſh to the end our people, as other natiõs do, might acquaint them ſelues with ſome part of this kinde, rather then with other friuolous diſcourſes, neither profitable to vſe, nor delectable to the vertuous, and well diſpoſed minde. This my ſlender endeuour I
dedicate

dedicate to your name right worshipfull M. Osbourne, to whom besides I am particularly beholdinge, your good fauouring of vertue and learning in certaine of my acquaintance of the best marke hath moued me to geue this signification howe readie learning is to honor her fauorers. she hath many daughters, and they be all knit in loue: betwixt thē there is neither enuie, nor iealousie: where one is honored and receiueth entertainment, there all congratulate without detraction: and euen as in a darke night one star breaking out of a thicke cloude, though it be but small, deliuereth a farre more cheerfull and comfortable light, then if it shone with many in a cleere euening: so this vertue hath the more grace, & beauty in you, insomuch as almost all such planets haue a long time either bene whollie eclipsed, or quite fallē out of their spheres, to the great discōforte of such as trauaile in this kinde of night workes, and busie thē selues at the lamps and are carefull to vpholde with perplexed studie the society of mankinde by learning and instruction. There be a fewe that shine with you, their honor grounded vpō vertue, shal stād for euer: the Muses and the Charites haue their names in perpetuall record: and I a seruant of theirs in their names performe this duetie vnto you in this sorte as I haue declared. Fareyou well: from litle S. Bartlemewes by Smithfield the 23 of May. 1586.

A louer of your vertue,

T. Bright.

TO HIS MELAN-
cholicke friend: M.

ALTHOVGH deare
M. your letter full of
heauines, and vncom-
fortable plaintes, hath in
such sort affected me, that (as it faireth
vvith a true harted friend) your affliction dravveth me into the fellovv-
ship of your mournefull estate. VVherby I am faine to call for such supporte,
as reason ministreth to vvisemen: and
am compelled as it vvere to put bit
into the mouth of my ouer vehement
affection: and giue checke as much as
my strength serueth vnto my passion
somevvhat in this behalfe vnruly. Yet
albeit our cases are not equall, in so
much as the griefe is not so sensible to
me as to your selfe, vvhome it hath (I

perceiue) entred to the quick, not onely of bodely sense: but hath passed deeper, and fretted the tender sinewves of the soule and spirite: yet I say, for asmuch as such is the gracious prouidence of our God, and the manifold graces of his bountifull hand vnto men, that scarce appeareth any calamity, but if time be taken and opportunitie laid holde on, helpe and release doth as readely present it selfe, to the comforte of such as trauaile vnder the burthen, as affliction is readie to charge them: and considering on vvhome this kinde of crosse is fallen: vpon a man exercised in the studie of pietie, and a practiser of the same, and one not ignorant of the preceptes of philosophie, vvherby vvordly men, and such as are destitute of the knovvledge of God, stay themselues in such cases, vvhich as it serueth them but slenderly and is but a readen staffe, to beare vp so heauy a burthen, being othervvise voide, and vnfurnished

of

of the heauenly grace, so may such philosophicall and humaine preceptes, and consideration of naturall causes, and euentes, stande him in steade, vvho resteth not vvholly there on, but leaneth vpon the maine pillar of Gods promises, of mercy and grace, and vvaighteth vvith patiēce the appointed time of his release. These considerations to be seene in you, giue me consolation and the rather inable me to comforte you my deare friēd, vvhose soule I perceiue pāteth vvith heat of that flame, vvhich most nigh you say in your feeling approcheth vnto those tormentes described vvher the vvorm dieth not and the fire goeth not out: vvhereof although you seeme presently to feele the anguish for a time; yet haue comfort and attend the happie issue, vvhich doubtles is your raising vp againe and more high aduauncement into the assurance of Gods loue and fauour. For as of all mettalls gold is tried vvith most

vehement heate, and abideth the oftenest hamering of vvorkemen for the refyning, vvhich being once fyned serueth for the seate of the Diamond, and for matter of precious vessels to the royall furniture of the tables of potentates and princes: so novv euen that heauenly refiner, holdeth you in this hote flame for a time, till being purified and cleared from that drosse of sinne vvhich cleaueth so fast, to our degenerat nature, you may make hereafter a more glorious vessell, for his seruice and honour of his heauenly maiestie. Your request is not onely that I should minister vnto you, vvhat my slender skill either in diuinitie or phisicke may afford, but that I vvould at large declare vnto you the nature of melancholie, vvhat causeth it, vvhat effectes it vvorketh, hovv cured, and farther to lay open, vvhatsoeuer may serue for the knovvledge thereof, vvith such companions of feare, sadnes

nes, desperation, teares, vveeping, sobbing, sighing, as follovv that mournefull traine, yea ofte times, vnbrideled
laughter, rising not from any comforte
of the heart, or gladnes of spirit, but
from a disposition in such sorte altered,
as by errour of conceite, that gesture is
in a counterfet maner bestovved vpon
that disagreeing passion, vvhose nature is rather to extinguish it selfe
vvith teares, then assvvaged by the
svveete breath of chearefulnes, othervvise to receiue refreshing: This your
request chargeth me vvith that,
vvhereto if my skill reacheth not, yet
my good vvill and prompt minde, both
in respect of your estate, vvhose griefe
I pitty and desire to mitigate, and the
complaintes of diuerse others also in
like case oppressed, dravve me, that
both they & you knovving the grouds
of these passions: vvhat parte nature
hath in the tragedie, and vvhat conscience of sinne driueth vnto: vvhat

difference betwixt them, how one
nourisheth another, how ech riseth,
and the seuerall meanes, both of pre-
uenting and cure of ech, the desperate
discouragementes, which rise vnto
bodie and minde thus afflicted may be
at the least mitigated, and some light
giuen to the soule, stumbling in the
darke midnight of ignorance, and refreshing to the comforteles hearte, distracted with a thousand doubtes and
pensiue thoughtes of dispaire: wherin
according to your request, I haue copiously entreated of these pointes, that
both you might be the more comforted
and satisfied by plentie of discourse, &
being a matter fitting your humor and
pertinent to your present estate, you
might haue wherewith to passe the
tedious time with more contentmēt.
Therefore as your griefe will giue
leaue and respitt thereto, you may here
know and learne that, which you
desire to know in this case, whereof
if

if by Gods blessing you may make vse to your cōfort, I shall ioye in my paines and you against other times of tryall, by this experience, may haue cause of more hope of release, and comfort in heauines, then through the terrour of this straunge affliction you presently feele.

THE CONTENTES OF
the booke according to the Chapters.

How diuerſlie the word melancholy is takē. Cap.1. pag.1.

The cauſes of naturall melancholie, and of the exceſſe thereof. Cap.2. pag.4.

Whether good nouriſhmente breede melancholie by fault of the bodie turning it into melancholie, & whether ſuch humour is founde in nouriſhmentes, or rather is made of them. Cap.3. pag.7.

The aunſwer to obiections made againſt the breeding of melancholicke humour out of nouriſhment. Cap.4. pag.10.

A more particular and farther anſwer to the former obiections. Cap.5. pag.22.

The causes of the increase & excesse of the melancholicke humour. Cap.6. pag 25.

Of the melancholicke excrement Cap.7.pag.31.

What burnt choller is, and the causes thereof. Cap.8.pag.32.

How melancholic worketh fearfull passions in the mind. Cap.9.pag.33.

How the body affecteth the soule Cap.10.pag.39.

Obiections against the manner howe the bodie affecteth the soule, with answer thereunto. Cap.11 pag.49.

A farther aunswer to the former obiections, and of the simple facultie of the soule, and onely organicall of spirit and bodie. Cap.12.pag.55.

Howe the soule by one simple facultie perfourmeth so manie and diuerse actions. Cap.13.pag.67.

The particular answers to the obiections

iections made in the 11.Chap. Cap. 14.pag.72.

Whether perturbations rise of humor, or not with a diuision of the perturbations.   Cap.15.pag.80.

Whether perturbations which are not moued by outward occasions rise of humour, or not: and how. Cap 16.pag.90.

How melācholy procureth feare, sadnes, dispaire, and such other passions.   Cap.17.pag.101

Of the vnnatural melācholy rising by adustion: how it affecteth vs with diuerse passions.   Cap.18.pag.110.

How sicknes, and yeares seeme to alter the mind, and the cause, & how the soule hath practise of senses separated frō the bodie. Cap.19.pag.116.

The accidentes which befall melancholie persons. Cap.20.pag.123.

How melācholy altereth the qualities of the bodie. Cap.21.pag.125.

How melancholy altereth those

actions which rise out of the braine. Cap.22.pag.129.

How affections be altered. Cap. 23.pag.132.

The causes of teares, and theire saltnes. Cap.24.pag.135.

Why teares endure not all the time of the cause: ard why in weeping commonly the finger is put in the eye. Cap.25.pag.148.

Of the partes of weeping: why the countenance is cast downe, the forehead lowreth: the nose droppeth, the lippe trembleth, &c. Cap.26.pag.123

The causes of sobbing, and sighing: and how weeping easeth the hearte. Cap.27.pag.157.

How melancholye causeth both weeping, and laughing with the reasons how. Cap.28.pag.161.

The causes of blushing, and bashfulnes, and why melancholy persons are giuē thereunto. Cap.29.pag.166.

Of the naturall actions altered by

melan-

melancholy. Cap.30.pag.173.

How melancholie altereth the naturall workes of the bodie: iuice, and excrement. Cap.31.pag.178.

Of the affliction of conscience for sinne. Cap.32.pag.184.

Whether the afflicted conscience be of melancholie. Cap.33.pag.187.

The particular difference betwixt melancholie, and the afflicted conscience in the same person. Cap. 34. pag.193.

The affliction of minde, to what persons it befalleth, and by what meanes. Cap.35.pag.198.

A consolation to the afflicted conscience. Cap.36.pag.207.

The cure of melancholie, & how melancholicke persons are to order them selues in actions of mind, sense, and motion. Cap.37.pag.242.

How melancholicke persons are to order thē selues in their affections. Cap.38.pag.249.

⁎ iiij

How melancholicke perſons are to order them ſelues in the reſt of their diet, and what choyce they are to make of ayer, meate, and drinke, houſe, and apparell. Cap.39.pa.257.

The cure by medicine meete for melancholicke perſons. Cap. 40. pag.265.

The maner of ſtrengthening melancholicke perſons after purging: with correction of ſome of their accidents.   Cap.41.pag.277.

A

A TREATISE OF MELAN-CHOLIE.

Chap. I.

Howe diuerslie the word Melancholie is taken.

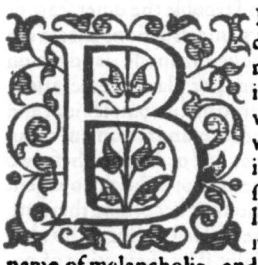EFORE I enter to define the nature of melancholie, & what it is, for the cleare vnderstãding of that wherein my purpose is to instruct you, it shall be necessarie to lay forth diuerse ma-ners of takinge the name of melancholie, and whereto the name being one, is applied diuerslie. It signifieth in all, either a certayne fearefull disposition of the mind altered from reason, or else an humour of the body, cõmonly taken to be the only cause of reason by feare in such sort depraued. This humour is of two sorts: naturall, or vnnaturall: na-turall is either the grosser part of the bloud or-

dained for nourishment, which either by abundance or immoderate hotenesse, passing measure, surchargeth the bodie, and yeeldeth vp to the braine certaine vapors, whereby the vnderstanding is obscured; or else is an excrement ordained to be auoyded out of the bodie, through so manie alterations of naturall heate, and varietie of concoction, hauing not a drop of nourishing iuyce remaining, whereby the bodie, either in power or substance may be relieued. This excrement, if it keepeth the bounds of his owne nature, breedeth lesse perturbance either to bodie or minde: if it corrupt and degenerate farther from it selfe and the qualitie of the bodie; then are all passions more vehement, & so out ragiously oppresse and trouble the quiet seate of the mind, that all organicall actions therof are mixed with melancholie madnesse; and reason turned to a vaine feare, or plaine desperation, the braine being altered in his complexion, and as it were transported into an instrument of an other make then it was first ordained: these two according to the diuersitie of setling, do ingender diuersitie of passions, & according therunto do diuerslie affect the vnderstanding, & do alter the affection, especially if by corruption of nature or euill custome of manners the partie be ouer passionate. The vnnaturall is an humour rising of melancholie before mentioned, or else from bloud or choler, whollie chaunged into an other nature by an vnkindly heate, which turneth these humours, which before were raunged vnder natures gouernment, and kept in order

Of Melancholie.

der, into a qualitie whollie repugnant, whose substance and vapor giueth such annoyance to all the partes, that as it passeth or is seated maketh strange alterations in our actions, whether they be animal or voluntarie, or naturall not depending vpon our will, and these are all which the name of melancholie doth signifie: now the definition and what it is. As the thinges be diuerse, so it also followeth the suite, and is likewise diuerse either of the humour or of the passion, and the humour being either a nutritiue iuyce or an excrement vnprofitable thereunto, I define the humor no otherwise then that part of that bloud which naturally of the rest is most grosse; and the excrement the superfluitie of the same; which if it putrifieth, bestoweth still the name of a farre diuerse thing both in temper & nature, called blacke choller. The melancholie passion is a doting of reason through vaine feare procured by fault of the melancholie humour. Thus brieflie & clearly do you vnderstand what the nature of melancholie is, and whereto the name is vsually applied: of which when I shall haue at the full to your contentment entreated, then will I satisfie the other part of your demaund, and lay open the consent and difference betwixt the conscience oppressed with sence of sinne and this naturall kinde before mētioned, and minister vnto you such heauenlie comfort and counsell as my slender skill will affoord, and such phisicke helpe as your present neede requireth.

A Treatise
Chap. II.
The causes of naturall melancholie and of the excesse thereof.

AS all naturall humours rise of nourishment, so melancholie being a part of bloud, from thence it springeth also. Whatsoeuer we receaue into the bodie for sustentation of this fraile life, consisteth of diuersitie of partes, being it selfe compounded, although to the outward viewe it seemeth to appeare vniforme: as bread, flesh, fish, milke, wine, beare &c. which shewe of vniformitie being taken away by the naturall furnace, which prserueth the liuely heate of euerie liuing thing, that outward resemblance vanisheth, and the diuersitie manifesteth it selfe: as we see gold or siluer, before it be proued with fire appeareth no other then all alike: but afterward is discouered by the burning crucible to be much otherwise; so fareth it with nourishments, whose diuerse partes are layd open by so manifold concoctions, and cleansings, and straininges, as are continually without intermission practized of nature in euerie mans bodie: no gold finer, more busie at the mine, or artificiall Chymist halfe so industrious in his laboratorie, as this naturall Chymist is in such preparations of all nourishment: be it meat, or drinke, of what sort soeuer. By this meanes the bloud which seemeth in all parts like it selfe, no egge liker one to another, is preserued distinct in all partes. The purest part which we call in comparison and in respect of the rest bloud, is temperate in qualitie,

OF MELANCHOLIE.

tie, and moderate in substance, exceeding all the other parts in quantitie, if the bodie be of equall temper, made for nourishment of the most temperate parts, and ingendring of spirits. The second is fleume, next to bloud in quantitie, of a waterie nature, cold and moyst, apt to be conuerted into the substance of purebloud if nature faile not in her workinge ordained for nourishment of moyster partes. The thirde is melancholie, of substance grosse and earthie, cold and drie in regard of the other, in quantity inferiour to fleume, fit nourishment for such partes as are of like temper. The fourth, choler, fierie, hote, and driest of qualitie, thinne in substance; least in quantitie, and ordained for such parts as require subtiller nourishment, and are tempered with greater portion of the fierie element. These differences nature hath so distinguished, that although in veine and place, they remaine linked together, yet in facultie, and vertue they are diuerse the one from the other: which as they fit the varietie of parts, bloud the temperate, and the rest such partes as haue like declining from temperate: so by the maruelous working of nature, these varieties of humours are entertained by nourishmentes inclining to like disposition: although no nourishment can be vtterly voide of all these parts, no not those that are counted most to encline to any one humour, as beefe, and veneson to melancholie: honie, and butter, to choler: and fish to fleume. Hereof riseth then this humour melancholie, euen from nourishments, as all the humours do;

A iij

and although not of such excellent vse; yet as necessarie for the maintenance of life and substance of the bodie as anie other; neither do these humoures fall into mans nature onely: but what soeuer liuing creature hath bloud can not be destitute of them as partes thereof, more or lesse according to their diuerse complexion. Thus then as man consisteth of partes requiring this diuersitie of foode, necessarie it was, and so ordained by God, such humours might aunswer in like varietie: and as humours are diuerse; so likewise the matter whereof they should be wrought could not be of one sort, and therefore all kinde of nature ordained for nourishment, affoord this choyce, some in greater scarsitie, this or that, to the end no state of body should complaine. Here you may moue a question not impertinent to the matter in hande; whether some bodies do not turne good nourishment, & of the purest sort into greater quantitie of melancholie, then other some, and whether that of nourishment which of it selfe would yeeld store of the best iuyce, by melancholicke or rather cold and drie disposition of the bodie, can so be altered as to faile of that store, wherewith by nature it is replenished, and in steede thereof yeeld this grosse, thicke, cold, & earthie humour, whereof I nowe discourse. Againe whether these humours are in such natures, as yeeld nourishment, and so by separation only after any Anaxagorian manner appeare, or rather are made as a stoole out of timber, bread of corne, wine of grape, &c.

CHAP.

Chap. III.

Whether good nourishments breedeth not store of melancholie by fault of the bodie: whether it turneth not into melancholie: and whether these humours are found in nourishments, or rather are made out of them.

THESE questions are not voide of probabilitie on both sides, which to the ende the truth may lye the more apparant, I will not stick to declare vnto you. It should seeme (as the objection importeth) that which before hath bene attributed to the kind of nourishment should rather rise of the bodie nourished, cōsidering how it altereth, which it embraceth for nourishment, as consider the earth it selfe, the mother & very nurse of all corruptible thinges, howe out of the same soyle, not halfe a foot betwixt the wholesome fruit and soueraigne medicine, both spring vp together with deadly poison: yea how in the selfe same creature what strange diuersitie of nature ariseth of the selfe same nourishment: as in the *pastinaca marina*, whose substance & flesh is wholsome to eat, & yet the taile carrieth a most deadly weapon, wherewith whatsoeuer is wounded, perisheth without recouerie, not by anie foraine tincture, but by the nourishment altered in that part into such a pernicious disposition. The same is also found in the flies *Cantharides*, whose bodie exulcerateth all parts, but especiallie the bladder, and is not inferiour to the chiefe poisons, contrarilie the wings help wherein the bodie hurted; which may be no small reasons of of doubt; whether the humors be found in nourishments, or rather are made by a certaine disposition of the bodie: as who would imagine, bloud could euer be made of yron; which notwithstanding, the Ostridges alter in such sort, as by no heate of fire, it can be sooner molten then it is digested in the stomach of that fethered foule? nowe nature digesteth nothing but to make vse of nourishment thereof: else whatsoeuer entreth into the bodie, passeth as it cometh, and hath no welcomming; but is refused as impertinent; nature bestowing no handling therof: more then a skilfull painter to counterfait the fashion of some excellent beautie, would dip his pensill in the mire, in steed of perfect colour. To these probabilities may be added, how some natures chaunge into a farre diuerse qualitie that which they haue receaued, then it stood by nature, as the family of Marsie in Italie, & Psillie in Lybia: which was so tẽpered, that they did without hurt sucke the poyson of vipers, and without perill did vsually hunt them: and so by necessary consequence to be gathered, that they did receaue nourishment by them. What soeuer entreth into the stomach, either is altered into familiaritie of nature: or else hauing an actuall power not hindered, altereth with repugnancie the nature which hath receaued it. If it altereth it wholly, then destroyeth it; if in part; then carieth it on the one part nourishing and alimentarie vertue, and on the other, a medicinable power; so it should seeme these Psillie, euen by vertue of nature made nourishment of that,

which

which to other is deadly poyson. Whereupon it may be gathered, that nourishments in some bodies haue not such power, as I haue said before; seeing they be made in certaine of poyson. The same may be declared in duckes and hennes, which feede vpon toads, notwithstanding their flesh we feed of with health, and strength, to our bodies; Quailes likewise feede of neesing powder seeds, and feldfares of hemlocke, tne one much approching nigh vnto, and the other famous by the Athenian executions. for most infamous poison. all which notwithstanding, their flesh is not refused at the tables of the most delicate and daintiest: hereby in apparance it seemeth that it skilleth not much, what meat is receaued in respect of sustaining this or that complexion; seeing that poysons may be made by vertue of concoction familiar nourishment: yea which is more auailable to vphold this matter, and straunge to consider of; it hath bene known and is recorded in credible historie, that some haue bene brought vp from their youth and alwayes haue bene sustained and fed with poyson; which being so, the nourishments of the bodie not onely receaue preparation by naturall concoction, by which they become that in deede & effect, which before they were in power & possibilitie: but seeme to be made out of whatsoeuer is receaued; where it findeth a nature of sufficient strength to frame it: and not (as it was wont to be sayd) Mercurie is not made of euery tree, so nature maketh euerie thing of any thing: not by Anaxagoras art, for then should breade containe really, corporally, and substantially flesh, bloud and bone, but by a power and vertue whereof the matter hath no part, more then the gold for the framing of a iewell partaketh of the goldsmithes cunning.

Chap. IIII.
The answer to the former obiections.

THESE shewes and semblances of truthes may seeme to ouerthrowe that which hath bene set downe as the ground and matter of humours, & lay it rather in the nature of the thing nourished, to transforme and assimulate whatsoeuer it hath receaued, though it be of neuer so straunge a qualitie: but as I haue set downe these obiections, to the end that truth being compared with vntruth may the better appeare by reason of comparison, so marke for your fuller satisfying in this point, howe yet nothing is hereby lost, but sufficiently it maintaineth it selfe: and by strength of reason, the only pillar of humane truthes it is vpholden. It was declared before how nourishments as of all other humours, so of melancholie, they affoord the matter, to the which nature applying her proper temper as an instrument, and practizing that skill which she hath learned of God, worketh out both humours and substance for preseruation and nourishment of our bodies; nowe that the earth within small distance affoordeth nourishment both to henbane & lettis, to hemlocke and the mallow, to poison and wholsome herbs;

that

that the same floure nourisheth the spider, and yeldeth honie to the bee, that the *pastinaca marina* carieth the instrument of death in her tayle, and wholsome foode in her substance, and all what hath bene before obiected from Cantharides; the Ostridges, Psilli and Marsi, neesing powder, hemlocke and toades, whereof wholesome birds do aduenture for nourishment, and from that virgine fed and sustained with poison sent vnto Alexander to infect him with hir companie: all I say that may out of these particulars encounter the former truthes, being considered and wayed, adde this thereunto (taking away nothing) that to the disposition of the matter, it is also necessarie, an outward skill and science in the worker concurre, whereby that matter may receaue conuenient forme agreable to the workers intention. For as it is impossible to make a rope of sande, so likewise hempe maketh it not without the art of the craftes man, who ioyning his worke with conuenient stuffe findeth the end of his labour: and as some workemen exceede other in skill & diligence and of the same matter, the worke either excelleth or wanteth according thereunto; in like manner the nourishment being all one, as it falleth to a nature of good or bad temper, weake or strong, bringeth forth nourishment, and excrement accordingly. Touching the earth it containeth in it inuisible seedes of all things in a maner, to which it storeth vp and importeth also food meet and conuenient: these seeds lye not distinct in place but in nature, no more then the partes of bloud which before I mentioned, so that although it were possible for hemlocke and the vine to grow in one bodie, and occupie one place, yet could not the proper nourishment to either be auoyded: such harmonie and agreement is there betwixt them in nature, and with such earnest desire doth the one affect the other. This then is the cause why life and death dwell so nigh together, and yet (as they are of the vehementest sort of aduersaries) without entercommunication. Euen so the bodie containeth partes linked notwithstanding in one communitie, of diuerse natures, which drawe out of the masse of nourishment that which is meete ech one for it self: which though it in apparance, & shew, semeth vniforme, yet containeth it diuersity, as the sundrie parts require: which diuersity being distinct in nature, & confused as it appeareth in one by the cloke & garment of an vniuersall forme; by natures Mechanical operation (the very patern of all arts, both liberall and seruile) is discouered & brought into an actuall substance consisting of his single & proper nature, which before had only a potentiall subsistence as members & parts haue in the whole. Which producing I vnderstand not a discouerie only, as by withdrawing a vaile, to shew that which lay behind it, but a generation and coupling of matter with the forme; which forme it bringeth not with it, but receaueth it as it were an impression from the part. So then, as euerie thing is not made of any thing in art; neither is foode ministred for all things in euerie thing in nature: but requireth

apt

apt preparation of matter, by naturall vertue to be appropriate to euerie part. Nowe if it be replied: this answer, as it may suffice against that which is obiected out of the earth, yet leaueth it doubt in the *pastinaca*, Cantharides and Psilli: by reason the matter of these things through natures working groweth more particular, & is not stored with such varietie (as I may so call them) of potentiall natures; whereby it might seeme the verie indiuiduall substance indifferently to subiect it selfe either for nourishment or poison: let the consideration of the earth carrie vs yet farther to the dissoluing of this knot also. True it is, that the particular nourishment containeth not so manie sutes, as the earth the nourisher of all things doth: yet it answereth in proportiō to the part which it hath to sustaine. So that the masse of bloud being the vniuersall soile, wāteth not for the relief & entertainment of al the mēbers of the bodie, choise of substance according to their variety. Hereof is the bone nourished, as hard as mettall: and the braine as tender as a posset curd: the kidneyes grosse and thicke: and the lights loose and subtile: the eye as cleere as cristall: and the splene as blacke and darke as inke. Now let vs apply this more particularly to Pastinaca, Cantharis, and the rest of that sort, The Pastinaca, substance, and fish, is nourished with that which in it selfe is wholesome, the fish being of the same substance or disposition; but so, that, that nourishment hath in it an execremental substance, which being considered alone though it be not yet poyson, hath in it a power, meeting with a former, to become of like hurtfull qualitie: which we see in execrements being permitted to putrifie and to degenerate of them selues, howe by corruption they become most daungerous; much more finding an actiue and liuely nature furnished with power as it were to animate and waken that which before lay dead in such matter: so Pastinaca hath a weapon geuen by nature soked with most deadly venome separated yet from the fish, and sticking on the one side of the middest of the taile, which is maintained with such a kinde of excrement, as being reiected in all the parts, findeth there impression and entertainment: not either that the fish feede of that poison (for nothing feedeth of excrement, appropriate to one part, or that wherewith that part, while it is excrement is nourished) as venimous, for then should such as feede of that fish be in perill, but being vnmeete to nourish or to haue place in the fish, is of temper, (by the altering of that part) apt to be conuerted into so venemous a nature, which is planted in the fishes tayle, not much vnlike to the growing of Misleto in a crab tree, whose natures do apparantly differ, seing the same Misleto groweth also in the oke & on the hauthorne: neither can anie with reason affirme, the Misleto is nourished with that which belongeth to the crab: for then would it not prosper in the oke destitute of his proper iuyce, but both the oke, the crab tree and the hauthorne, certaine of them, and in certaine places, hauing a superfluiti: meete for that vse, the seed of that misle being

OF MELANCHOLIE.

being there and embracing that humour, riseth vp into such a diuerse plant as we see; which yet according to the diuersitie of place, varieth in vertue, for that only of the oke we vse and accompt auaileable against the falling sicknesse & esteeme the other of small value. Nowe if it be demaunded, why then groweth not the misle on the earth, which hath more plenty of such iuice, and greater choyce? it may be thus aunswered: although the earth affoordeth entertainement for all things, yet it doth it diuersly, to some immediatly, to other some by meanes, as the earth ministreth iuyce to the grasse and herbe of the common field, it nourisheth mutton, & we feed thereof; who if we should attempt to be releeued by the herbe, it would yeeld vs but thinne fare. This iuyce of the earth is altered into another nature in the herbe, that herbe into flesh, and flesh of that kinde chaunged into the substance of our bodies, which first as it sprung vp from the earth, so by it is it releeued. So the misle draweth from the earth, by meanes of the tree wherewith it prospereth, indued now with other forme, & made more familiar vnto it, by the preparation of the tree. And this I take to be the cause why certaine things will not growe on the earth, but in other natures: and why graffes yeld more pleasant fruit then carnels, by reason the stocke giueth the crude and rawe nourishment of the earth a farther ripening, and euen as it were chewing it vnto the sion graffed: so to conclude this aunswer; the Pastinacas venome is ministred by an excrement, which carieth an aptnes to be couerted into poison:and such poison as that part is able:therof to engender, neither being such before in the Pastimaces nourishment, nor in the substance of the fish, nor as excrement; but after it is conuerted thereinto by that barbed weapon; which the fish reuēgeth within her tayle. Whereby it is euident, that not only of poyson, but of any humor beside, the aptnes of the matter (whereof some be grosser, and some passe more alterations) it is necessary also there shoulde concurre in the place nourished, an altering vertue; and as such assimilation is necessary, in like manner an apt matter may not be to seeke, fit for such generation. Wherefore Melancholie is not made of euerie part of good nourishment, but of such parte, as hath a token of fellowship with the same Melancholie: and more or lesse as the bodie is more or lesse apte, together with aptnes of the matter to make that conuersion. Touching the Ostridge which may seeme to turne yron into blood and so into flesh: we are rather thus to esteeme, that although the Ostridges nature doth intend nourishment by the yron; yet doth it no more nourish, then stones doth chickins, & hennes which are dissolued in their mawes. How thē (say you) & why doth it dissolue yron? by a contrary vertue which respecteth all thinges alike, that are receiued: whereby the stomach becommeth the most Catholicke parte in all the bodie, carying a more indifferent affection to whatsoeuer is receiued then anie part beside, which in the first concoctiō regardeth not so much it self as other partes,

OF MELANCHOLIE.

partes, for whose sake it is ordayned, as it were, the Cooke not respecting this or that sorte of nourishment or foode, but applying it selfe alike generally to all that hath not a resistance in nature and a counterpower of poyson, which alwayes altereth and is not altered. Else could it not so easily embrace both hote and cold, sower and sweete, fat and leane, moyst and drie, of all bougetts (as a certaine Poet sayth) in that respect the straungest; by this vertue the Ostridges hauing a verie thick and fleshie mawe, whereby it is furnished with store of a naturall heate dissolueth by a kinde of putrefaction, the yron; which if it yeeld anie nourishment, the stomach findeth benefite thereof in the blood, wherwith it is nourished, if none, it passeth all into excrement and so is voyded as vnprofitable, except it may be thought more likely in reason, that the Ostridges enioyeth some parte of nourishment, thereby passing it into blood, or at the least that the stomach receiueth a kinde of comfort and contentment, which commonly it is taken to do by the nourishment it containeth as the Cooks appetite may be satisfied for a time by smelling of the rost, which if it faire so with the stomach there is then reason sufficient of such digestion which the fowle worketh not by the excesse of heat, but by a certaine temper apt for the work, for no heate of fire in longe time is able to doe that which the Ostridge mawe doth speedelie by a certaine corruption of that which it digesteth. Carying as it were a kinde of *Aqua fortis* in the mawe, rather then anie heate of *Etna*, if we

B

take it that the fowle hath some parte in the bodie, whose turne the common officer, the stomach serueth, agreeing to the nature of some substance contained in the yron, & that conueyed into the blood, and from thence drawen to that part, wherof it is affected: or it hath an Alementarie vertue common to diuerse partes. Be it so, yet therefore no consequence of reason can inferre, that nature respecteth not anie aptnes of matter: for in a manner al things of the earth hath some thinge Alimentarie and pasturable for all liuing creatures, which may euidētly appeare by cōparing of nature. The earth which we plow and till and labour with hard and wearie hand is altogether mynerall, which is the generalleſt nourishment of all: now if one nature among so manie millions be found in yron to sucke forth that vertue, no maruell seing all creatures which require releefe of foode, by certaine degrees and former apparations, pertake of the same: then seing the Mineralls feede the Vegetalls, and the Vegetalls the Animalls; let the experience of the Oſtridge satisfie vs in this which reasoñ misliketh not, that euen a nutritiue iuice for some sorte of Animall may be foúd in yron, and yet so, that (notwithstanding) not all things are of like aptnes for such vse, neither in generall as blood, nor in particular, as the more speciall food belonging to ech parte deriued from the blood. And thus my friend *M.* to passe the tedious time with you, you haue my opinion to this obiection. As for the ſtraunge nature of that kinde of people or famelie called

Marſi

OF MELANCHOLIE.

Marsi and *Psilli*, we may thus reasonably coniecture, that either they had a nature of stronger temper, then the ordinary sorte, by which it was able to maister that poyson and all other; or else by the custome of vsuall feeding on the flesh of aspes and vipers, which they did vse, they grewe into such familiarity with the poyson, as the serpentes themselues, which nature had with such poison so armed, and this rather then that infamous refuge of propriety of substance, which is asmuch to say, as we knowe not. This custome was also the only cause why the yong maid nourished with poyson faired with it as with other victuall: for of purpose she was nourished from her infancie therwith, that she might by frequēting the Kinges companie destroy him with infection, which poyson being but an accidentary thing, by custome is vanquished of a naturall & essentiall vertue. That poyson is but accidentall and not essentiall, it appeareth by that in diuers kindes, it is not in all of the same sorte, nor alike in all partes of such natures, as we count venemous, as the wings of Cantharides and the bodies so contend in nature, that the one helpeth where the other harmeth: the weapon of Pastinaca and the fish, the Scorpion and his stinge, the vipers bitte and vipers flesh, the base and foundation of Triacle, the shrewmouse and her selfe dissected and applied to the wound: which all argue the poyson not to be equallie mixed, and therefore not essentiall: againe in some places Scorpions are not hurtefull, in some spiders, in other some aspides, the which if their nature

B ij

did consist of poyson, then could they not be otherwise, neither receiue alteration by soile, neither is this in animalls onelie, but also in vegetalls, as in Persea, in Hemlockes, in Napellus in the Vgh tree which in other some places carie with them certaine and assured perill, and in other some are vtterly harmeles. This custome being begunne in infancie, made a greater familiaritie betwixt the damsells nature, & the poyson, which as in ciuill manners it is more flexible in youth thē in processe of yeares, so the disposition of nature fareth in like sort, which most hartely embraceth that wherewith it is first acquainted, but you wil say; how could it haue first accesse and be entertayned of nature, to whome it is so repugnant. Thus we are to iudge in the case, that they which first practised this straūge kinde of nourishing, by litle and litle assayed nature, and now and then gaue harte therunto by counterpoyson preseruatiues, and so at the last, being encouraged, and farther strengthened, it was able to ouercome that parte of the poyson; which of it selfe was deadly and turne the other into familiar nourishment, which by reason of acquaintāce through custome, her nature brake which if it had ben all poyson, then as it had bin whollie & vnfit matter of nourishment, so could shee not without daunger haue borne it one howre: whereby it is manifest, that with natures arte an apt matter of producing of nourishment must needes meete for her maintenance. That which Cantharides offereth of doubt, may be sufficiently resolued by that which hath bin said

of

OF MELANCHOLIE.

of Paſtinaca. The quailes feeding of Hēlock, & the other of neeſing powder, moue more difficult queſtions, ſeing they make the poiſon holeſome nouriſhment to themſelues & yeeld their bodies, daintie diſhes to our tables, notwithſtāding their poyſoned foode: Whereby it ſhould ſeeme, that poyſon it ſelf, where a nature fitteth, therewith may be matter of holeſome nouriſhment, for the ſatiſfying of which obieƈtion, we are to conſider euerie parte of that we take for nouriſhment, is not alimentall but parte excrement, and that the greateſt parte, as it appeareth by ſo manie alterations, and purginges, which the foode ſuffereth, before it be receiued of the partes of the bodie for proper nouriſhment. ſo therfore; theſe birdes are not ſuſtained with that which is poyſonfull in their foode, but alter it firſt, and then paſſe it into ſuperfluous excrement; their ſubſtance being vtterly voide of the ſame, and ſo becometh vnto vs holeſome: verie well: but how is their nature able to vanquiſh that which is poyſon: ſeing it is not receiued of vs without preſent daunger? Diuerſe reaſons thereof may be alleadged, firſt, it is not poiſon vnto them, as we ſee ſome kindes of Aconites to kill dogges, ſome Leopardes, and ſome wolues, and not offenſiue to our creatures: then, that it may be by exceſſiue heate of the mawes of ſuch birdes, then cold poyſon of Hemlock receiueth ſufficient alteration to keepe of the perrill of poyſon. Whereto may alſo be added, the reaſon of Galen, that becauſe the vaines & paſſages of thoſe birdes are ſtraighte, the poyſon before it assaileth the hart in the way receiueth sufficient alteration; especially Hemlock being so cold poyson, and therefore flowe of passage in respect of it selfe, and shutting vp, and straightening of poores, by which it passeth: so to conclude this probleme, we see the sentence standeth yet sure, that nourishments are the matter of all humors, and by consequence of Melancholie, and although natures wonderfull arte appeareth in making (as it may seeme in apparance) one contrary to another, yet doth it not so in deede, but alwayes desireth conuenient matter to practise her naturall acte vpon: and thus much to the obiections, now to the questions themselues.

Chap. v.
Touching the questions propounded in the end of the second Chapter.

THvs much hath bene said to the obiectiōs, now let vs declare at large to your fuller satisfying, what I iudge most agreable to the truth in the questions: and first, whether some bodies do not turne good nourishment, and of the purest sort into greater quantitie of melancholie, then other some? which question if we consider parted, it may more clearly be decided, that is, first whether the same nourishment be not turned into more or lesse plentie of melancholie in other bodies? then, whether by anie qualitie of temper, good and pure nourishment may yeeld an humour melancholicke? To these questions
first

first I aunswer affirmatiuely, yet not impairing of the former truth set downe. For all kinde of nourishment as it in part altereth the bodies, so is it againe of them more altered then it altereth, whereby melancholicke persons of the self same nourishment frame vnto them selues that which to them selues is agreeable: else could there be no nourishment without this altering vertue. Why then (say you) it riseth not of the nourishment, which was not melancholicke, but of the nature nourished. Not so, for no nourishment is so pure, that altogether it is voyd of melancholicke matter, for then could it not be nourishment: but notwithstanding it hath greater plentie of good nourishment then of grosse and melancholicke, the similitude of nature refuseth the one, and embraceth the other: whereupon riseth this difference in nourishment, the vitall being alone. The second part of the former question, receaueth the same answer with the first, because no nourishment is so pure but it partaketh little or much, with some part of melancholie. For I do not take it, that the part maketh the nourishment melancholicke, which carieth no disposition thereunto: but lusteth after that in the masse of victualles, wherewith it hath greater familiaritie, which to a melancholicke bodie is of an impurer disposition, refusing that would serue more fitly for a better tempered complexion; euen as we see oft by experiéce that the good complexion may be replenished with melancholicke bloud: which appeareth by opening a vaine, and yet the parties bodie nou-

B iiij

rished, (as the beautie of colour doth declare) with that which is pure, which melancholicke bloud rose of euill choice of diet, rather then through fault of complexion: nowe that part of nourishment, that is pure cannot be altered in substance into another, whereto it carrieth no proportion: by mixture it may be defiled, and become impure, but neither can it be altered into that, wherewith it hath no community, more then grosse, melancholicke, and earthy nourishment can by any art of nature become aëry, moderate and pure: I meane the self same part of nourishment: for so might all things in deede rise of euerie thing, which would turne the excellent varietie of naturall things into vnitie. As for Anaxagoras imagination of breeding things by separation onely, this kind of diuerse matter, which we require in nourishment euerthroweth it, neither are we to thinke generation of nourishment to be no other but as art worketh vpon her subiect, for there is there no nature produced, distinct in substance and essence, but by an accidentall qualitie only produced by art. And thus lest I be ouer tedious in this point, you haue my answer to the questions and obiections before made concerning the nature of nourishing and preparation of humors, and hitherto that hath bene sayd, respecteth only melancholie, as it is an humour in the bodie apt for nourishment of certaine partes, more disposed to that, then to any other portion of the bloud besides, nowe touching the cause of increase and excesse of this humour.

CHAP.

Chap. VI.
Of the causes of the increase and excesse of melancholicke humour.

IT was declared that the quantitie of melancholic should be least in the iust téper of bloud of all the other parts, sauing choler, which naturall proportion and rate when it exceedeth, then is the bodie turned into a disposition melancholicke by humour: although the cóplexion for a time hold entire, which long can not endure, more then the nature of that damsel which was nourished with poyson, kept her ingenerated complexion: but nature acquainting it selfe by moments and degrees with such kind of humour, and hauing no choice of better, is faine at length to embrace that, which otherwise more gladly it would reiect. The causes of excesse of this humour are diuerse, and all (except it be receaued from the parent) spring from fault of diet: and although chieflie meates and drinkes do yeeld matter to this humour, yet besides the complexion inclining to such temper, this matter is increased by perturbatió of mind, by temper of aire, and kind of habitation, and that humour which otherwise would yeeld a nutritiue iuyce, of the best sort, by this occasion is turned into these dregges of melancholie. Here first I will declare vnto you, such nourishments as are apt to engender those humours, that in this present state you nowe stand in, oppressed therewith, knowing which they are that minister matter to this grosse iuyce, you for your more speedie recouerie auoide them, and with choice of better, alter that which is amisse into a more cheerfull qualitie. Nowe all nourishmentes that offende vs, either do it by their owne nature, or by some accidentarie cause befalling vnto them, and likewise whatsoeuer becommeth vnto vs melancholicke. But that you may more easilie vnderstand from whence all sorts of nourishments are taken, I will set downe vnto you in a short viewe, the kinds of them all, and in euerie kind note vnto you, that which of the owne nature is melancholicke. You knowe all nourishmentes are either meate or drinke: meates are taken either from vegetables or animalls: the vegetables either minister vnto vs nourishment them selues, or their fruit onely, & they are either of trees or herbs: of trees, the tender buds are eaten, which because we do litle vse to feed of, I passe ouer farther mention. Of herbes we either feede of the root, or such partes as rise therefrom, and those roots are either round or long, of neither sort do I remember anie greatly to be eschewed as melancholicke, except rape rootes & nauewes. Such parts as rise from the root, are vsed while they be tender and young, or else sprung vp at the full, of these kinds, coleworts, beete, and cabages only ingender a melancholicke iuyce. The fruites of vegetables are either of trees or herbes: of fruits of trees, quinces rawe, medlers, seruices, dates, oliues, chesnuts and acornes are all melancholicke: fruites of herbes, are either graine or of other sort, and those are either corne or pulse:

Of Melancholie. 27

of corne, sodden wheate is of a grosse and melancholicke nourishment, and bread especiallie of the fine flower vnleauened: of this sort, are bag puddings, or pan puddings made with flour, fritters, pancakes, such as we call Banberie cakes, and those great ones confected with butter, egges &c. vsed at weddings, and howsoeuer it be prepared, rie and bread made thereof, carieth with it plentie of melancholie. The pulses are wholy to be eschewed, of such as are disposed to melancholie: except white pease: fruites of herbes of other sort then graine are purest from melancholicke excesse. And thus of vegetables you vnderstand, which you haue in this melancholicke respect to be auoyded. The food which we take from the animals, is either from them selues, and from certaine of their wholesome excrements. Such as yeeld them selues are either of the earth, or of the water: those of the earth haue great diuersitie of nourishment in their seuerall parts, which are either spermaticall, and those of white colour: or sanguine, of colour redde and bloudie. The spermaticall partes may well be discharged of melancholicke iuyce, as rather enclining to fleume. Of the sanguine partes, some are the brawnie parts, which compasse the bones, and are ordayned for voluntarie motion, called muscles: or else are of the inward partes, and are of them selues destitute of motion. The muscles which are subiect to most motion, as of the leggs, yeeld more melancholie, then partes which haue more rest. Of the inwardes, the milt is altogether melancholicke, & so the kidneyes, the liuer, the heart, and with them, all the carnels. Bloud is melancholicke, and whatsoeuer dish thereof is made. Nowe all nourishments taken from the earth, are either beastes, or foule. Of beasts; these are of melancholike persons to be eschewed: porke, except it be yong, and a litle corned with salt, beefe, ramme mutton, goate, bores flesh, & veneson: neither is mutton of anie sort greatly commended of Galen. Of foule, some be water foule, and some land. The water foule are not of melancholicke persons to be tasted, except the goosewings. The land foule which are melancholicke are these: feldfares, thrushes, sparowes, martins, turtles, ringdoues, quailes, plouers, peacockes &c. and these haue you to eschew of nourishments of the earth. Those of the water are fish: & either of the salt water and sea; or of the fresh water. Such as are of the sea, are either of the monsters of the sea; or such as more properly are to be called fish. The mōsters are ceals purposes, & such like: which all breed vnwholesome & melancholicke nourishment. The fish of the sea are either shell fish, or destitute of such defence. Of shell fish, some are of harder shels, as oysters, periwincks, muscles, cockles, & such like: of which ranke, the oyster carieth with it least suspition of melancholy. The softer shell or crustie are cray fish, the crab, the lobster, the pūger, & such of the riuers like to these &c. which all neede not to be excepted vnto you in order of your diet. Such sea fish as carie no armor of shels, are ether those, that haunt the rocks: or

other

other parts of the sea. The rocke fishes are most apt of all maner sea fish, for melancholicke persons: as the gilthead, the whiting, the sea perch &c. Such as haunt other places, are either keepers of the depth; or aprochers nigh the sand & shore. Of such as keepe the depth, either they haue the pooles: or other places of the depth. Of the poole fishes, I remember not any greatly to be auoyded in choyce of your diet. Of such as frequent other places of the depth, these are melancholicke: the dragon of the sea, in forme like an eyle: the cuckoe, ling, anie salt fish, thornbacke, and skate. Of such as approch the shore, I knowe none greatly to be auoyded. Fresh water fish, and of the riuer: the lampray, and the tench, haue most plentie of melancholie. And these are nourishments taken from the parts of the animals: now their works are either excrements, & superfluities of their humors, or other kinds of workes. Of the first sort, are milke from the beast, and egges from the foule: which the spawne of fish in a maner resembleth: milke, and what soeuer is made thereof, is to be eschewed of melancholic persons: as cheese, curdes, &c. the spaunes, as roes of hearinges, are to be eschued of you, as nourishment of melancholie: else I take none of that sort greatly to be feared in that respect. Of other works of animals then excrements, we feed only of honie, which hath no melancholy dispositiō at al. Of drinks, eschue red wine, and what soeuer liquor, beare, ale, or cider, is not cleere, & well fined: as also if it be tart, and sower. Hitherto haue you hearde of nourishmentes, which of thier owne nature are to be eschued; nowe of those that by some accident, and not of them selues are melancholicke, as if they be too olde, and verie leane: or be long kept: or ouer much salted: whereby they become the drier and harder, you are to refuse them. Likewise if in the dressing of the nourishment, it be ouermuch baked, or rosted, it is to be eschued. To these belong salt fishe, beefe, and bacon, and redde hearringes, hard cheese, and old. Of drinkes, newe wine, beare or ale: and on the contrarie part, ouer stale, and sower, are to be eschued: and of sauces, those that be sharpe, as veriuyce, aliger, or beareger, vineger, are chiefly to be auoided of melancholicke persons. Thus do you vnderstand howe to vse your choice in meates, and drinks: and what to shunne, as breeders of this thicke, blacke, and melancholicke humour. Besides these, the aire thicke and grosse is fit to entertaine this humor: so that fumie, marrish, mislie, and lowe habitations, are hurtfull to persons disposed to melancholie: likewise if it be dimme & dark. Wherfore the houses, & habitations of that sort, are most vnmeete for such persons. These hitherto are all such outward things melancholick: whatsoeuer else breedeth melancholie, is a disorderly behauiour of our owne parts, in such actiõs as belonge to the gouernement of our health. This behauiour, is either in actions of motion: or in order and manner of rest. Our motion, is either of mind, or bodie. Of actions of the minde, ouer vehement studies, and sadde passions, do alter

good

good nourishmentes into a melancholicke qualitie; by wasting the pure Spirites, and the subtill-
est parte of the blood: and thereby leauing the
rest grosse and thicke. In like sorte do exercises
either wholly intermitted; or turned into an excessiue labour, and wearying of the bodie: the
one causing the blood to be thicke through setling: and the other, by spending the bodie ouermuch, & drying it excessiuely. Such also as giue
themselues to inordinate sleepe, therby further
the encrease of melancholicke humours. And
these are all the causes, whereby the matter of
that humour is supplyed; and the blood being of
it selfe good, is altered into that iuice, whereof
you complaine of abundance. Now if to these,
you adde a nature of it selfe disposed thereto, &
a splene not able, either for feeblenes, or obstruction, to purge the blood of superfluitie of that
iuyce, then haue you all that may be said of the
causes of this humour, keeping within the compasse of nourishment.

Chap. VII.
Of melancholicke excrementes.

THE melancholicke excrement is bredde of
melancholie iuyce, drawen of the milte out
of the liuer, by a braunch of the porte vayne,
wherewith being nourished, it reiecteth the rest
as meere excrementall; and voydeth parte, into
the mouth of the stomach, to prouoke appetite,
and hunger; and passeth the other parte in some
persones, by hemerode vaynes into the siege: It

aboundeth there when it is hindered of such passage as nature requireth; or else by feeblenes of the parte, it is not able, either to suck the melancholie from the blood, or discharge it self into those passages, which nature hath therto ordained. This member, of the whole bodie is the grossest, and euill fauouredst to be held, blacke of colour, and euill sauorie of taste: and giueth a manifest experience of natures desire, alwayes to couet that, whereto it is most like; and so faireth the splene better with those muddy dreggs, then it would with purer and finer blood; which if it should be offered to other parts, they would abstaine: except great want forced them to take anie parte thereof. These are the causes of naturall melancholie, both iuyce, and excrement: It remaineth next, to shewe, what that humour is, which riseth of this, or anie else, corrupted, called also by the name of melancholie.

Chap. VIII.
What burnt Choler is, and the causes thereof.

THAT kinde of melancholie, which is called *Atra bilis*, riseth by excessiue heate of such partes, where it is engendred or receiued, wherby the humour is so adust, as it becommeth of such an exulcerating, and fretting qualitie, that it wasteth those partes, where it lighteth; this most commonly riseth of the melancholie excrement before said, and diuerse times of the other thicke parte of blood; as also of Choler, and
salt

salt fleame: which take such heate, partely by distemper of the bodie, and partly by putrefaction that thereby a humor riseth, breeding most terrible accidentes to the minde, and painefull to the bodie: which the melancholicke and grosse bloud, doth more forcibly procure: in that that anie heate, the grosser the substance is, wherein it is receaued, the more fiercely it consumeth: whereupon the seacole giueth more vehement heate, then charcole: and the cole then the flame: and a cauterie of hote yron, then a burning firebrand. Otherwise choler being by nature of the hotest temper, carieth with it, more qualitie of heat then the other: but by reason the substance of the humor is more subtle and rare, the lesse it appeareth: &, as the heat of a flame in comparison of the other, more speedily passeth. Hitherto haue I declared vnto you all the kinds of melancholy, and causes of ech of them: hereafter you shall vnderstand, how they worke these fearefull effectes in the mind, wherby the hart is made heauie, the spirites dulled, the cheerfull countenance altered into mourning, and life it selfe, which the nature of all thinges most desireth, made tedious vnto persons thus afflicted.

CHAP. IX.
Howe melancholie worketh fearefull passions in the mind.

BEFORE I declare vnto you how this humor afflicteth the minde: first it shall be necessarie for you to vnderstand, what the familiaritie

C

is betwixt mind and bodie: howe it affecteth it, and how it is affected of it againe. You knowe, God first created all things subiect to the course of times, and corruption of the earth, after that hee had distinguished the confused masse of things, into the heauens, & the foure elements. This earth he had endued with a fecunditie of infinite seeds of all things: which he commaunded it, as a mother, to bring forth, and as it is most agreable to their nature, to entertaine with nourishment, that which it had borne, & brought forth: whereby when he had all the furniture of this inferiour world, of these creatures, some he fixed there still, and maintaineth the seedes, till the end of all things, and that determinate time, which he hath ordained, for the emptying of those seedes of creatures, which he first indued the earth withall. Other some, that is to say, the animals, he drewe wholly from the earth at the beginning, and planted seede in them onely, and food from other creatures: as beasts, and man in respect of his body: the difference only this: that likely it is, mans body was made of purer mould, as a most pretious tabernacle and temple, wherin the image of God should afterward be inshrined: and being formed as it were by Gods proper hand, receaued a greater dignitie of beauty, and proportion, and stature erect: therby to be put in mind whither to direct the religious seruice of his Creator. This tabernacle thus wrought, as the grosse part yeelded a masse for the proportion to be framed of: so had it by the blessing of God, before inspired, a spirituall

thing

Of Melancholie.

thing of greater excellencie, then the redde earth, which offered it self to the eye onely. This is that which Philosophers call the spirit: which spirit, so prepareth that worke to the receauing of the soule, that with more agrement, the soule, and bodie, haue growne into acquaintance: and is ordained of God, as it were a true loue knot, to couple heauen & earth together; yea a more diuine nature, then the heauens with a base clod of earth: which otherwise would neuer haue growen into societie: and hath such indifferent affection vnto both, that it is to both equally affected, and communicateth the bodie and corporall things with the mind, and spirituall, and intelligible things, after a sort with the bodie: sauing sometimes by vehemencie of eithers actiō, they seeme to be distracted, and the minde to neglect the bodie: and the bodie and bodilie actions common with other creatures, to refuse as it were for a moment that communitie wherby it commeth to passe, that in vehement contemplations, men see not, that which is before their eyes: neither heare, though noyse beat the ayre and sound: nor feele, which at other time (such bent of the minde being remitted) they should perceaue the sence of, with pleasure or paine. This spirit is the chiefe instrument, and immediate, whereby the soule bestoweth the exercises of her facultie in her bodie, that passeth to and fro in a moment, nothing in swiftnesse & nimblenesse being comparable thereunto: which when it is depraued by anie occasion, either rising from the bodie: or by other meanes, then

becometh it an instrument vnhansome for performance of such actiós, as require the vse therof: and so the minde seemeth to be blame worthy: wherein it is blamelesse: and fault of certaine actions imputed thereunto: wherein the bodie and this spirite are rather to be charged, thinges corporall and earthly: the one, in substance, and the other in respect of that mixture, wherewith the Lord tempered the whole masse in the beginning. And that you may haue greater assurance in reason of this corporall inclination of spirit, consider how it is nourished: and with more euidence, it shal so appeare vnto you. It is maintained by nourishments, whether they be of the vegetable, or animall kind: which creatures, affoord not only their corporall substance; but a spirituall matter also: wherewith euerie nourishment, more or lesse is indued: this spirit of theirs, is (as similitude of nature, more nighly approcheth) altered more speedely, or with larger trauell of nature. Of all things of ordinarie vse, the most speedy alteration is of wine: which in a moment repaireth our spirits, and reuiueth vs againe, being spent with heauinesse: or any otherwise whatsoeuer, our naturall spirites being diminished: which bread, and flesh, doth in longer time: being of flower passage, and their spirites not so subtile, or at least fettered as it were in a more grosse bodie: and without this spirit, no creature could giue vs sustentation. For it is a knot, to ioyne both our soules and bodies together: so nothing of other nature can haue corporall coniunction with vs; except their spirites
with

with ours firſt growe into acquaintance: which is more ſpeedily done a great deale, then the increaſe of the firme ſubſtance : which you may euidently perceaue in that we are ready to faint, for want of foode; after a litle taken into the ſtomach of refreſhing, before any concoction can be halfe reformed, the ſtrength returneth, and the ſpirit reuiueth, and ſufficient contentment ſeemeth to be giuen to nature: which notwithſtanding, not fully ſo ſatisfied, prepareth farther the aliment of firme ſubſtance, and ſpirits of purer ſort, for the continuall ſupply of thoſe ingenerate, for ſence & motion, life & nouriſhment. Nowe although theſe ſpirites riſe from earthly creatures; yet are they more excellent, then earth, or the earthie parts of thoſe natures, from which they are drawne; and riſe from that diuine influence of life, and are not of them ſelues earthie: neither yet comparable in purenneſſe & excellencie, vnto that breath of life, wherewith the Lord made Adam a liuing ſoule, which proceeded not from any creature, that he had before made, as the life of beaſts and trees; but immediatly from him ſelfe, repreſenting in ſome part the character of his image. So then theſe three we haue in our nature to conſider diſtinct, for the clearer vnderſtanding of that I am to intreate of: the bodie of earth: the ſpirit from vertue of that ſpirit, which did as it were hatch that great egge of Chaos: & the ſoule inſpired from God, a nature eternall and diuine, not fettered with the bodie, as certaine Philoſophers haue taken it: but handfaſted therwith, by that golden claspe of the spirit: whereby, one, (till the predestinate time be expired, and the bodie become vnmeet for so pure a spouse) ioyeth at, and taketh liking of the other. Nowe as it is not possible to passe from one extreme to an other, but by a meane; and no meane is there in the nature of man, but spirit: by this only the bodie affecteth the mind: and the bodie and spirits affected, partly by disorder, and partly through outward occasions, minister discontentment as it were to the mind: and in the ende breake that bande of fellowship, wherewith they were both linked together. This affecting of the minde, I vnderstand not to be any empairing of the nature thereof; or decay of any facultie therein; or shortning of immortality; or any such infirmitie inflicted vpon the soule from the bodie (for it is farre exempt from all such alteration): but such a disposition, and such discontentment, as a false stringed lute, giueth to the musician: or a rough and euill fashioned pen, to the cunning writer; which only obscureth, the shew of either art, and nothing diminisheth of that facultie, which with better instruments, would fully content the eye with a faire hand; & satisfie the eare with most pleasant and delectable harmonie. Otherwise the soule receaueth no hurt from the bodie; it being spirituall, and voyde of all passion of corporall thinges; and the other grosse, earthie, and farre vnable to annoy a nature of such excellencie.

CHAP.

Chap. x.
How the bodie affecteth the soule.

IN this sorte then are you to conceiue me, touching those actions, which the bodie seemeth to offer violence to the soule; in that no alteration of substance, or nature, can rise there from, nor anie blemish of naturall facultie, or decaye of such qualities, as are essentiall vnto the soule: otherwise, might it in the end perish, and destroy that immortall nature; which can not by anie meanes decaie, but by the same power which created it. But thus onely doe (as I may so call them) passions force the soule; euē through the euill disposed instrument of the bodie, they depraue the most excellent and most perfect actions, whereto the soule is bent in the whole order of mans nature, and by corruption of the Spirites, which should be the sacred band of vnitie, cause such mislike, as the soule, without that mediation, disdaineth the bodies longer fellowship, and betaketh it selfe, to that contemplation, whereto it is by nature inclyned; and giueth ouer the grosse, and mechanicall actions of the bodie, whereto, by order of creation, it was allotted in the earthly tabernacle. But you wil say vnto me, experience seemeth to declare a further passion of the soule from the bodie then I mention: for we see what issues, bodelie thinges, and the bodie it selfe driue our mindes vnto: as some kinde of musicke, to heauines; other some to chearefulnes; other some to compassion; other some to rage; other to modestie; and other to wantonnes:likewise of visible thinges, certayne sturre vs to indignation and disdayne;and other to contentednes,and good liking.In like manner certaine natures take inward, moue vs to mirth; as wyne;and other to heauines;some to rage,furie and frensie;and other some to dulnes & heauines of spirite : as certaine poysones in both kinds do manifest these passions vnto vs;besides such as rise of our humours bredde in our owne bodies; which may be reasons, to one not well aduised,so to mistake these effectes of corporall thinges,as though the soule receiued farther impression, not onely in affection, but also in vnderstanding, then I haue vnto you mentioned: for satisfying of you, in which doubtes,you are diligently to consider,what I shall declare, concerning the seuerall actions of bodie, soule and spirite, and how, each one of these performeth their actions;which must be kept distinct,for better vnderstanding of that I shall hereafter in this discourse lay open vnto you. And first, concerning the actions of the soule:you remember how it was first made by inspiration from God himselfe,a creature immortall, proceeding from the eternall;with whome there is no mortality. The end of this creation was, that being vnited to the bodely substance, raised and furnished with corporall faculties from the earth,commō with other liuing creatures, there might rise a creature of middle nature betwixt Angels,& beastes, to glorifie his name.This the soule doth, by two kindes of actions:the one kinde,is such as it exerciseth, seperated from the bodie; which are contem-

OF MELANCHOLIE.

contemplations of God, in such measure as he is by naturall instinct opened vnto it, with reuerent recognisaunce of such blessinges, as by creation it is endued with. Next vnto God, whatsoeuer within compasse of her conceite is immortall, without tediousnes, or trauell, and with spirituall ioye incōparable. These actiōs she is busied with in this life, so long as she inhabiteth her earthly tabernacle; neither in such perfection, nor yet so freely, as she doth seperated, and the knot loosed betwixt her and the body, being withdrawē, by actions exercised with corporall instrument, of baser sort. These are the other kinde which the soule, by the creators law is subiect vnto, for the continuance of the creature, and maintenance of the whole nature, with dueties thereto belonging; animall, vitall, naturall; and whatsoeuer mixed, requireth iovntly. ll three; as this corporall praising of God for his goodnes, and praying vnto him for necessities, releeuing our brothers want, and defending him from wrong; with euerie ones seuerall vocation, wherein his peculiar charge lyeth; whether it be in peace, or in warre; at home, or abroade, with our countrymen, or with straungers; in our owne famelies, or with our neighbours; whether it be superiority of commaudement, or duety of obediēce: which differ in degree, as they be nigher, or farther of the actions peculiar to the soule; or communicate more, or lesse with them. If you say vnto me; how commeth it to passe, that the soule being of so single, and diuine a nature, as the creation manifestly sheweth, intermedleth with so grosse actions, as are common, not onely with bruite beastes; as sense, motion and appetite; but euen also with natures of farre inferiour condition, as plantes, and mineralls: whereby it seemeth, that, either the soule is not of such excellency, as in truth it is; or else that our nature consisteth of three soules, to which seuerall faculties, and actions are alotted. By deeper consideration of the nature of the soule, this obiectiō may be easily aunswered. The soule, as the substance therof is most pure, and perfect, and far of remoued from corruption; so it is endued with faculties of like qualitie, pure, immortall and answerable to so diuine a subiect; & carrieth with it, an instinct science, gotten, neither by precept, nor practise; but naturally therewith furnished; whereby it is able, with one vniuersall, and simple facultie, to performe so many varieties of actions, as the instrument, by which it performeth them, carrieth an apt inclination thereto: as the brayne being an instrument of conceite, it therewith conceiueth: the eye to see, it seeth: the eare to heare, it heareth: and so the instrument of smelling, and taste, wanting nothing of their naturall disposition, the soule smelleth with, & discerneth tasts: which otherwise disposed, it can not shewe that ingenerate instinct, by outward senses, the faculty yet notwithstanding remayning entyre and vntouched: I say the facultie, and not faculties. For if we plant so many faculties in the soule, as there be outward, and inward actions performed by vs, it certainely could not be simple, but needes must receiue varietie of composition; to

aunswere

Of Melancholie. 43

answer so many faculties, as we see insensible creatures; which as they worke diuersly, so haue they diuerse varieties of substance, of which sort among many other is Aloe, Rhubarb, and diuers simples, that with one parte of their substance, loose, and open; and with the other stoppe and staie; the same also is sensible in colewortes and Cabages; and in the substance of shell fishes: whose decoction looseth the bodie, and procureth soliblenes; their substance being of a quite contrary operation: which riseth of a diuerse tépered substance in one nature, compounded of such varietie, whereof as the soule together vniforme, is voide, so can it not possesse any variety of facultie. This if it seeme straunge vnto you, considering the diuerse sorts of actions, and the vnlikelines of performance of so many, and so diuerse; I will as I may in a matter, so difficult, & aboue the reach of any similitude of visible creature (except it selfe) only by comparison, make the assertion more plaine. Compare the skill of painting, with this simple and vniforme faculty of the soule: the faculty is simple and one, and yet cold Apelles therewith vse both the grosse, & the small pensill; he could draw a line cuident to the eye a farre of, and so subtle, that scarse might it be discerned nigh at hand; he could applie himselfe by his vniforme faculty, to all the parts of Venus beauty: otherwise must it of necessitie follow, that so many instrumentes of painting as he vsed, so many kinds of lines as he could draw, and so many partes as he could counterfet; the eye, the nose, the mouth, &c, so many sundry faculties of painting had he; which to a man not destitute of the facultie of reason, must needes seeme most absurd. The same appeareth in the art of musick, which being attayned vnto, but one facultie, yet is it the same: in all the kindes of moodes & variety of tune, and time: although the practise be diuerse. Euen so, the soule hath a faculty one, single, and essentiall, notwithstanding so many and sundry partes are performed, in the organicall bodies, as we dayly put in practise: neither is it hereof to be gathered, that the soule affordeth no mo actions, then there be instruments: for both her proper actions, require none, and the other common with the bodye, by diuerse vsing and applying of the same instrumēt, are manifold and sundry, and the more sundry, the more generall the instrument is, and pliable, to diuerse vses: euen so, as the soule, in organicall actions, vseth one and the selfe same instrument to chaungeable offices; likewise being separated from the body, although the faculty be one, it also exerciseth of her selfe, without instrument, from one faculty, diuers dueties. And thus haue you my opiniō touching the actions of the soule, either considered, seperate: or cōioyned with the body: and being ioyned therunto, such as it exerciseth of it selfe: or by those organicall meanes as the body affordeth: it remaineth, next to entreate of the spirite, and of the bodie, with their seuerall actions. Of such organes, as the soule vseth for instrumentall actions, some are of substance, & nature most quick, rare, and subtile: other some grosse, slow, & earthy

OF MELANCHOLIE.

thy, more, or lesse. The subtile instrument, is the spirite: which is the most vniuersall instrument of the soule, and embraceth at ful, so farre as bodely vses require, al the vniuersall faculty, wherwith the soule is indued, and directeth it, and guideth it, vnto more particular instruments, for more speciall and priuate vses, as to the eye, to see with; to the eare to heare; to the nose to smell; to the bowells, stomack, and liuer, to nourish, to the heart, to maintaine life: and to other partes, to the end of propagation: this is all performed by the selfe same, one, and single spirite. If you demaunde whereof this spirite is made? I take it, to be an effectuall, and pregnāt substāce, bred in all thinges, at what time the spirit of the Lord did, as it were, hatch, and breede out all liuing thinges, out of that Chaos mentioned in the Genesis; which Chaos, as it was matter of corporall, and palpable substance to all thinges: so did it also, minister this liuely spirit vnto thē, diuerse and seuerall, according to the diuersitie of those seedes, which God indued it withall: to some more pure: to other some more grosse, according to the excellency of the creature, and dignitie of the vses, wherto it is to be employed: from this power of God, sprange the spirite of man, as I take it, raised from the earth, together with the body, whereby it receiued such furniture, and preparatiō; as it becommeth a lodging, for so noble a gest, except it may seeme more likely, to be infused, and inspired, into the bodie, with that breath of life, which was the soule of man, at what time, god had first made his corps, of the mould of the earth; which I for certayne reasons here following am moued to make doubt of. First, although it be an excellent creature, and farre excedeth the grosse substance of our bodie; yet is it baser, then to be attributed to so diuine a beginning, as from God immediatly; especially considering it hath not only beginning; but perisheth also: to which cōdition, nothing that proceedeth from God in such special manner, as the soule did, can be subiect vnto. Againe, we see this spirit maintained, and nourished by the vse of earthly creatures; and is either plentifull, or scanteth; as it hath want, or abundance of such corporall nourishment. Now to drawe the originall ofspring of the spirite of man from God, were in a maner to drawe from him the spirit of all other things, wherewith that of man is releeued: which can not be accompted to flowe from that breathing of God; both seeing the Scripture pronounceth it, as peculiar to the soule of man: and otherwise, should they be not inferiour in that respect, to the soules of men; which by nature, are set vnder his feete; and in all respects are farre inferiour vnto him: that I mentiō not, too nigh approching the maiestie of God: which without impaire thereof, admitteth not so nigh, the accesse of the nature of inferiour creatures; honoring mankind therwith only of all his visible workes. Thus then, as I take it, both the spirite had his first beginning, and is of such nature as I haue declared; and serueth for these vses. I know commonly there are accompted three spirits: animall, vitall and naturall:

turall: but these are in deede, rather distinctiõs of diuerse offices of one spirit; then diuersity of nature. For as well might they make as many as there be seuerall parts, and offices in the bodie; which were both false, & superfluous. Next ensueth the nature of the bodie, and his seuerall instruments, with their vses; which my purpose is here so farre to touch, as it concerneth the vnderstanding of that ensueth of my discourse: leauing the large handling thereof to that most excellent hymne of Galen. Touching the vse of the parts: the bodie being of substance grosse, & earthy; resembleth the matter whereof it was made: and is distinct into diuerse members, and diuerse parts, for seuerall vses required, partly of nature, and partly of the humane societie of life: whereupon, the braine is the chiefe instrument of sense, and motion, which it deriueth by the spirit before mentioned,' into all the partes of the bodie; as also of thoughtes, and cogitations, perfourmed by common sense, and fantasie: and storing vp as it were, that which it hath conceaued in the chest of memorie: all which the braine it selfe with farther communication exerciseth alone. The hart is the seate of life, and of affections, and perturbations, of loue, or hate, like, or dislike; of such thinges as fall within compasse of sense; either outward, or inward; in effect, or imagination onely. The liuer the instrument of nourishment, & groweth: & is serued of the stomach by appetite of meats and drinkes; and of other parts, with lust of propagation: & as the hart, by arteries conueigheth life to all partes of the bodie: so the liuer, by vaines distributeth her faculties to euery member; thereby the body enioying nourishment, & increase, serued with naturall appetite, whereby ech part satisfieth it selfe with that, which therto is most agreable. And these actions are bodily performed of the soule, by employing that excellent, and catholicke instrument of spirit, to the mechanicall workes of the grosse, and earthy partes of our bodies. Thus then the whole nature of man, being compounded of two extremities, the soule, and the bodie: and of the meane of spirits: the soule receaueth no other annoyance by the bodie; then the craftes man by his instrument: with no impeach, or impaire of cunning: but an hinderance of exercising the excellent partes of his skill: either when the instrument is altogether vnapt, and serueth for no vse: or in part only fit; wherby actions, and effects are wrought, much inferiour to the faculty of the worker: & as the instrument is of more particular vse, so is the soule the lesse impeached: and as more generall, so yet more hindered: both from varietie, and perfection of actiō: as the hart, more then the liuer: and the liuer, more then the braine: the stomach more then the rest of the entrailles: and all publicke parts, more then priuate: of which sort the spirit being disordered, either in temper, or lessened in quātitie, or entermixed with straunge vapours, and spirits, most of all, worketh annoyance, and disgraceth the worke, and crosseth the soules absolute intention: as shall more particularly appeare

peare in the processe of my discourse: which that it may yeeld vnto you full aunswer of such doubts, as may arise vnto you, and make question of the truth of this point: I will my selfe set downe such obiections, as may encounter the credit thereof, and aunswer them, I hope, to your satisfying.

Chap. xi.
Obiections against the former sentence, touching the maner how the soule is affected of the bodie: with answer thereto.

THE obiections which seeme to enforce vpō the body farther power ouer the soule, then to withstand the organicall actions, are such, as are taken from the dispositiō of our bodies, both in health, and in sicknesse. In health, we see how the minde altereth in apparance, not onely in action, but also in facultie: both in that some faculties spring vp, which before were not: and those through occasions of chaunge of the body either more perfect, then otherwise they haue bene, or would be. This appeareth in age, and in diuerse order of diet, and custome of sensuall & sensible things. First touching age and yeares: we see in childhoode, howe childish the minde beareth it selfe, in facultie incomparable to that which afterward it sheweth: as the vnderstanding dull: the wit of blunter conceipt: memorie slipperie: and iudgement scarse appeareth. The body growing vp, and attaining at length the height of his increase, all these giftes, more and

D

more growe vp therewith: and (euen as the bodie) get maturitie, and strength, which is the perfection in their kind. Againe the bodie passing the point of his vigor and virilitie of age, turneth all the wits and sage counsels, into more then childish doting: by which alterations and chaunges, in apparance the mind both suffereth detriment, and againe receaueth greater ability of facultie. Neither is this only brought to passe through processe of years: but also it may seeme that certaine faculties, which before were not, at a season of age, put forth, and aduaunce them selues, which before gaue no countenaunce of shewe: and, except we shall make nature keepe idle holy day, in them were not at all: as the facultie of propagation, of all naturall sorts, one of the chiefest: which, if we say it slept, as it were in the mind, or waited a day: it should seeme verie ridiculous, that nature should be furnished so many yeares with a facultie, which it should put in practise so long after: especially considering how particular faculties attend onely vpon single and particular vses, and haue no other employing. If it were not before, then either should the mind be imperfect at the first, wanting some part of the furniture: or else should it seeme to rise of the temper of the bodie: either of which, attribute more vnto the bodie, then of right thereto belongeth: and calleth in question the immortalitie of the soule: except you will say, it is a facultie, whereof the soule hath no part, being common with brute beastes: which carieth with it these absurdities. First, this facultie

cultie muſt needs haue her ſeate, either in ſoule or bodie: if it be not in ſoule, then in bodie: if in bodie; then ſhould the inſtrument poſſeſſe the facultie, which is as one would attribute the facultie of the harmonie to the harp, and the writing to the pen, and not to the ſcriuener: eſteeming the skilfull harps, and skilfull pens, which are dead inſtruments, and haue no being of motion in them ſelues. Now middle ſubiect is there none, whereto this facultie ſhould fall, except we will vainly, and againſt reaſon and philoſophie admit mo ſoules then one in our bodies. Againe, to place any facultie otherwiſe then of diſpoſition, and aptneſſe, in the bodie, without the ſoule, were to diſturb the vniforme gouernment, and that œconomicall order, wherby our nature is ruled; in placing mo commanders then one. So we ſee, howe age, and courſe of times affect the bodie, not only by alteration of facultie, as it ſhould ſeeme, but alſo, by breeding new. Nowe the order of life, region, and diet, ſeeme to preſſe the matter further: and as it were, to turne the mind about, with euerie blaſt of corporall chaunge. We may obſerue the nature of mariners, occupied in the ſea ſurges, who haue their maners not much vnlike framed, tempeſtuous and ſtormie: likewiſe the villager, who buſieth him ſelfe about his plow, and cattell only, hath his wits of no higher conceit: butchers acquainted with ſlaughter, are accópted therby to be of a more cruell diſpoſition: and therefore amongſt vs are diſcharged from iuries of life & death: theſe experiences maintaine the quarel,

D ij

against the vnmoueable, and vnchaungeable facultie of the soule, whereof I haue before made mention. Howe region, and aire make demonstration of the same, the comparison of the gentle, and constant aire of Asia, with the sharpe & vnstable of Europe, doth declare vnto vs: wherby the Asians are milde, and gentle, vnfittte for warre, and giuen to subiection: the Europians, naturally, rough, hardie, stearne, right martiall impes, and harder to be subdued, and raunged vnder obedience: and of the same region, such people as inhabite places barren, open, and dry, and subiect to mutabilitie of weather, are more fierce, bolder, sharp, and obstinate in opinion, then people of contrary habitation. Neither hath diet lesse part in this case of affecting the soule, then the rest: for we see, howe the chearfull fruite of the vine maketh the hart merie, and giueth (with moderation vsed) an edge of wit, and quicknesse to the spirits: and those nourishmentes that are moyst, grosse, and not firmely compacted, aggrauateth the vnderstanding, and maketh the conceit blunt, and disableth much the faculties of the minde: which a thinner, drier, and more subtile foode doth entertaine. To these obiectiós may be added, what alteration of minde, diuersitie of complexion, & excesse of the foure humours; choler, fleume, bloud, and melancholie do procure, not only to the affections, as sanguine cheerefulnesse, melancholicke sadnesse, fleume heauinesse, & choler anger: but to the wits, and such faculties as approch nigher to the soueraigne partes of our

nature,

nature, the mind it selfe: as choler procureth rashnesse, and vnaduisednesse, with mobilitie & vnstablenesse of purpose: melancholie contrarily, pertinacie, with aduised deliberatiō: sanguine simplicitie: and fleume flat foolishnesse: and these are, so farre as my memory serueth me, all that is wonted to be obiected from the state of our bodies, being in health, against the perpetuall, & immoueable tranquillitie of our minds, and immortall, vnchaungeable, and incorruptible faculties therof: which all in the next Chapter, I will satisfie with full aunswer: nowe a fewe wordes touching the perturbarions, and alterations through sicknesse: and so will I ende this Chapter, and in the next proceede to seuerall aunswers. I my selfe haue obserued it diuerse times, not onely perturbation of minde to arise by certaine diseases, whereby it fancieth, and reasoneth disorderly: but some faculties euen amended by the same (neither faculties of base action) as for the eye, to see clearer after an inflammation: and conuulsions to be helped by agues: and in feuers, the hearing more quicke then before, and the smelling more subtile: and in phrenticke persons, the strength doubled vpō them: but also euen apprehension more perfect, and memory amended, and deliuerance of tale more free, and eloquent without all comparison: which are actions of the greatest organicall practises of the mind: in such sort that I haue knowen children languishing of the splene, obstructed, and altered in temper, talke with grauitie and wisedome, surpassing those tender yeares, and their iudgement carying a maruelous imitation of the wisedome of the ancient, hauing after a sorte, attained that by disease, which other haue by course of yeares: whereupon I take it, the prouerbe ariseth: that they be of short life, who are of wit so pregnant: because their bodies do receaue by nature so speedie a ripenesse, as thereby age is hastened, through a certaine temper of their bodies, either the whole, or in some animall part: which ripenesse as in other creatures, it easily yeeldeth to rottennesse, so in our nature, that speedy maturitie hasteth to declination, and sooner decayeth. Thus for your full satisfying, I haue called to minde such obiections, as do chiefly giue checke vnto that which I haue propounded touching the passions which the body chargeth the soule with: now shall you vnderstand the solution, & clearing of these doubts. If you will descend into the consideration of the effectes of poisons in our natures, as of henbane, coriander, hemlock, nightshade, and such like, they will giue greater euidence vnto that which these obiections import: by which the mind seemeth greatly to be altered, & quite put beside the reasonable vse of her ingenerate faculties during the force of the poysons: which being maistred, or at least rebated, by cōuenient remedies, it recouereth those gifts, wherof it was in daunger to suffer wracke before: and if it be true which Plato affirmeth, that cōmon wealths alter by change of musicke, what stablenesse shall we account in the mind, w̄ is in this sort subiect to euery blast of chaunge?

CHAP.

Chap. XII.

The aunswere to the former obiections and of the simple facultie of the soule and only organicall of spirite, and bodie.

THESE doubtes before mentioned, I will answere in such order as they were in the former chapter obiected: beginning with those alterations, which the soule seemeth to sustaine from the bodie, while it enioyeth health, and good state of all his partes: of which sorte age & yeares first inferre against vs. For the generall aunswere whereof, as also for the rest, we are to hold two pointes, as vnfallible, before mentioned: the one, is the simple faculty of the minde: and the other, the organicall vse only of the body and spirite: which two groundes, before I enter into the particular disciphiring of the obiections, I will first establish by reason, and thē apply them to the particular solutiō of that which hath bene obiected. First, the simplicitie of the nature of the soule, more simple then the heauens, argueth vnitie of facultie: seing all simple thinges by nature reiect mixture and composition, and whatsoeuer tendeth to pluralty. For, whatsoeuer is more, is diuerse, diuersity, simple thinges embrace not, neither doth diuersity of nature admit so nigh copulation, as to settle themselues in the selfe same simple, & vniforme subiect: which if they refuse to do, what shall we iudge then of will, and appetite repugnant to reason: and will sometime at variance with animall appetite? how can these so contrary faculties concurre in one single nature? That, simple thinges receiue neither cōtrarietie, nor diuersity, the consideration of the whole sort of dissentanie, and disagreeing things, wil make the matter manifest. All of that kinde are either such as we call diuerse, or opposite: diuerse, whose disagreement is most gentle, haue notwithstāding such strife, that they meete not in the selfe same subiect at any time: as beauty, and wisedome, riches, and honestie: which haue their diuerse roomes in the same generall nature, and do not one farther encounter the other. The other, haue one single subiect, if they be of accidentary natures, or qualities: and there one expelleth the other: enduring no society: as vertue, vice, liberality, couetousnes, and prodigality: black, blew, yellow, and greene: light, darknes, &c. And these are at perpetuall warre, & admit no truice day, no not for a minute, & so, because they will needes possesse the same place, expel ech other, and are in Logick tearmed, Opposites. Now thē whatsoeuer the soule simple, indiuiduall, & without mixture or composition giueth entertaynement of disagreeing natures, must of necessity fall into one of these: that is, to the opposite or diuerse. The opposite require, their owne times, and will not accord in the same subiect at once, except you will accompt relatiues of a milder disposition, & more sociable then their fellowes which notwithstanding by the diuerse respect, are as farre disioyned as the rest. Now then, if we hold that the minde hath diuerse faculties, then of necessitie must there be in the same

minde

minde diuersity of subiect: which if ther be, then is the simplicity thereof turned into multiplicity of substance, and composition of nature: a disposition contrarie both to the manner of the beginning of the soule void of mixture, and that immortall perpetuitie, wherewith it is induced. Peraduenture it may seeme straūge, and repugnant to the nature of thinges diuerse, to d.sleuer them of subiect, seing softnes and whitenes, white and heate, and such like, being diuerse enter into the same subiect: as in snoe, the one and the other in molton leade, or hote yron: which doubt, because it serueth for proofe of this vnity of faculty, I will lay open, and make playne vnto you. Of all things subiect to corruption, the elementes are most simple, which being diuersly mixed, yeeld the variety, we see of all compoūd thinges vnder heauen: these haue ech of them, but one quality: fire hote, ayer moist, earth dry, and water cold, if they should haue twayne, then must they needes either entercommunicate, or two quallities concurre with the first matter: entercommunication is there none: for then should they not be the elements of other things seing they should be elemēts one of ech other: two qualities make superfluities in the mixed, which nature eschueth in all her worke: then superfluitie would be here in that there should in the compound be found a drynes of fire, and the like of earth: a coldnes of the earth, and the like of water: and so in the heat of fire, & ayre: which were more then neede: seing such quallities are sufficiently imparted to the compound by one.

Now if the elementes which after a sort receiue composition of a grosse matter and forme, do admit no diuerse quality, much lesse doth the minde of a more pure beginning, and simple substance, reiect the same. But how then commeth it to passe, that a cole is black and hard, & chalk harde and white, in the same parte throughout, if diuersities settle no nigher together? yea very well notwithstanding. For compounded things, though they make one nature, yet are they not by reason of composition in all partes alike, neither are the elements so confused in the mixture but in all partes they may be found distinct by their qualities simple or compound: which qualities although they be commonly attributed to the whole, yet properly and cheefely, belong they to the elementes whereof the whole cōsisteth: so that in one nature, diuersity of subiect is to be considered. Example shall make it plaine: The heate of pepper riseth of the fiery element; the drynes and solidity, of substaunce which it hath of the earthie. In Rhubarb the purging vertue riseth of the subtle substance, & the strengthening facultie of the grosse and earthy. Chalk is white of the aiery moisture which it is endued with: and hath his hardnes of a earthie drynes. The rose her rednes of a certaine temper of single moistnes, concocted with heat: and her smell, of an aierie moistnes mixed with an earthy drynes, attenuated with heate, and vertue of the fiery element? So we see diuerse thinges, which seeme to fall into one vniuersall nature or subiect, the matter being more narrowly

Of Melancholie.

rowly vined, betake them to their owne subiect, proper and peculiar vnto themselues, and only by communicating their substaunce with the whole, endue it also with like qualities. But you will say: if the elements haue but one qualitye (which first was affirmed to the mainteynance of single faculty) then is not the element of fire dry, nor of water moist, nor of aire warme. True: neither are they of their owne natures such: but that which is in fire beside heate, is only an absence of moistnes: in the earth accompted cold, is an absence only of heate: in the rest likewise, and not an ingenerate quallity: more then heauen may be said to be moist, because it is not dry or hote, because it is not cold: which indifferently refuseth all such kinde of quallity. Now an absence of one quallity, is not straight waye an inferring of the other: but only in priuants, wherof the one is a meere absence, and of that contrary only, which naturally should be present: as blindnes is not rightly said of a stone, though it see not at any time. In the elemetary qualities, it is not so: but they are all quallities, importing a presence: because they adioyned to the first matter of thinges, are the only formes of elementes: now absence formeth nothing, and priuants are alwayes contrary to forme and nature: It appeareth then, that elements which are lesse simple then the soules of men are endued but with one faculty, and that diuerse things require a diuerse peculiar seat, which being taken vp in such natures as will abide mixture, seeme as though they were of the whole mixed, when as but after a sort only they are so to be accōpted. These two pointes being sufficiently proued establish euidently the simple and vniforme faculties of the soule: For hereby it is most manifest that by reason of the simple nature thereof, it cannot beare any mixture, or be support of diuerse thinges: neither that diuerse will so neighbour it together, as to dwell in one indiuiduall subiect. Then seing that they which of al the disagreers, least disagree, will not so nighly be linked. neither can any diuersity of faculty in the minde, in a nature so simple, and impartible be coupled together, where ther is no disagreemēt of substance, nor dissent of mixture, but euery parte like the whole, and ech like other. Againe these pluralities being essentiall, can be but one: seing essence is not many, and nature alwayes farre vnlike the sword of Delphos; which serued for diuerse vses, euer employeth one to one, and not to many: otherwise wāt should enforce her, which (she abounding with sufficiency) refuseth in all her actions. Moreouer being in euery part like it selfe, and ech parte like other, no dissimilitude can arise by distinction of faculty. Accidentall if they be: then is the minde in daunger of loosing all faculty, which it cannot do seing it is subiect to no force, but of God himselfe that made it. Now whatsoeuer naturall faculty in any thing fadeth, it is by reason the thing first fadeth which enioyeth that faculty: else would they alwayes continue: wherefore the minde being euerlasting, and exempt from chaunge and corruption, her faculty is also essentiall, and of like

perpe-

perpetuity: I neede not yeeld reason why contrary faculties, or such as we call disparates in logicke, can haue no roome in a nature so simple as the soule is, both in respect of the repugnance within themselues, and vnitie of the subiect: seing such as are diuerse only refuse that cohabitation and neighbourhood. Thus much shal suffice to proue the simple faculty of the soule: it followeth to proue the spirite and body to be wholly organicall: by organicall I meane a disposition & aptnes only, without any free worke or action, otherwise then at the mindes commãdement: else should there be mo beginninges & causes of action then one, in one nature: which popularity of administratiõ, nature will none of, nor yet with any holy garcicall or mixt: but commandeth only by one soueraintie: the rest being vassals at the beck of the soueraigne commander. The kindes of instruments are of two sorts: the one dead in it selfe, and destitute of all motion: as a saw before it be moued of the workman, and a ship before it be stirred with winde, and hoised of saile: the other sorte is liuely, and carrieth in it selfe aptnes, and disposition of motiõ: as the hound to hunt with, and the hauke to fowle with, both caried with hope of pray: the hand, to moue at our pleasure, and to vse any other kinde of instrument or toole. The second sort of these twaine, is also to be distinguished in twaine, whereof the one obtaineth power in it selfe, and requireth derection only, as the beast, and fowle aboue mentioned: and the other not only direction, but impulsion also from an inward vertue, and forcible power: as the motion of the hand, and the variety of the hand actions do most euidently declare. Of these three kinds of instruments, I place the spirit and bodie both to the mind, as the saw or axe in the workmans hand, or to the lute touched of the Musician (according to the sundry qualities & conditions of the instruments of the body) in the thirde sort; but so, as the spirit, in comparison of the bodie, fareth as the hand to the dead instrumentes. Of the first sort they are not, because they partake of life: of the second they may not be, because of them selues they haue no impulsion, as it appeareth euidently in animall and voluntarie actions, and (although more obscurely to be seene) in such as be called naturall. For the spirit being either withdrawne from the outwarde parts by vehement passiō of griefe, or ouer prodigally scattered by ioy, or wasted by paine, the outward partes not only faile in their sense and motion, but euen nourishment & growth therby are hindered: and contrarily, though the spirit be present, except the part be also well disposed, not only feeling is impaired, & such actions as require sense and motion, but also concoction and nourishment. Againe, the spirit it self without impulsion of minde lieth idle in the bodie. This appeareth in animall actions more plainly: as the mind imploying vehemently the spirit an other way, we neither see that is set before our eyes, nor heare, nor feele that which otherwise with delight, or displeasure, would vehemently affect vs. In naturall actions and parts, it is more obscure:

obscure: either because the spirit can not be altogether so separated by the order of nature, being rooted so in the part, or because the verie presence of the soule in an organicall bodie, without further facultie or action, carieth the life withal, and is not subiect to arbitrement and will: as the royall estate of a Prince, moueth silence, reuerence, and expectation, although there be no charge, or commaundement therof giuen, nor such purpose of presence: so life lieth rather in the essence, or substance of the soule, giuing it to a fit organed body; rather then by any such facultie resident therein. except we may thinke that lesse portion of spirit serueth for life onely, then for life, sense, and motion, & so the parts, contented with smaller prouision thereof, are entertained with life, though sense and mouing require more plenty. But howsoeuer this be obscure in naturall actions, the mind transporting the spirits another way by sudden conceit, study or passion: yet most certaine it is, if it holde on long, and release not, the nourishment will also faile, the increase of the body diminish, and the flower of beautie fade, and finally death take his fatall hold: which commeth to passe; not onely by expence of spirit, but by leauing destitute the parts, whereby declining to decay, they become at length vnmeete for the entertainement of so noble an inhabitant as is the soule, of stocke diuine, of immortall perpetuity, and exempt from all corruption. Then seeing neither body, nor spirit are admitted in the first, or second sort of instruments, they fall to the third kinde, which being liuely, or at the least apt for life, require direction, and also foreine impulsion: foraine, in respect of them selues, destitute of facultie, otherwise then disposition: but inward and domesticall, in that it proceedeth from a naturall power, (resident in these corporall members) which we call the soule: not working as ingens, by a force voide of skill and cunning in it f.lfe,& by a motion giuen by deuise of the Mechenist: but farre otherwise indued with science, & possessed of the mouer: as if Architas had bin him selfe within his flying doues, & Vulcanne within his walking stooles, and the mouing engine as it were animated with the minde of the worker, therein excelling farre all industrie of art. For here the natural Apelles painteth as well within as without; and Phydias is no lesse curious in polishing the entralles, and partes withholden from the viewe, then in garnishing the outward apparance, and shew of his frame: and which is yet more, here the crafts man entreth him selfe into all the parts of the worke, and neuer would relinquish the same. Although we place the spirit and body in the third kind of instruments, yet is there great oddes, betwixt these two. For the spirit answereth at full all the organicall actions of the soule, & hath in it no distinction of members: the body is of more particular vses, compounded of sundry parts, ech of them framed of peculiar duties, as the mind and spirit employeth them. The spirit is quicke, nimble, and of maruelous celeritie of motion; the body, slow, dull, and giuen to rest of it selfe: the spirit the verie hand

hand of the soule; the body & bodily members like flailes, sawes, or axes in the hand of him that vseth them. For as we see God hath geuen vs reason for all particular faculties, and hand for all instruments, of pleasure, of necessitie, of offence, of defence, that thereby, although man be borne without couering, without teeth, without hoofe or horne, only with tender nailes, and those neither in fashion, nor temper fit for fight: yet he clotheth him selfe, both against the tempest warme, against force of weapon with coate of steele, and maketh vnto him selfe weapons of warre, no tush, no horne, no hoofe, no snout of elephant in force comparable thereunto: so the spirits of our bodies, and this hand of our souls, though it be but one, yet handleth it all the instruments of our body: and it being light, subtile, and yeelding, yet forceth it the heauiest, & grossest, & hardest parts of our bodies, chewing with the teeth, and striking with the fist, & bearing downe with the thrust of shoulder, the resistance of that which standeth firme, and containing alone the force of all the members: seeth with the eye, heareth with the eares, vnderstandeth organically with the braine, distributeth life with the hart, and nourishment with the liuer, and whatsoeuer other bodely action is practised. This hand is applied to the grosse instrument, and the effect brought to passe, yet not absolutely of it selfe, but by impulsiō of the mind, which is placed the only agent, absolute and soueraigne not onely in respect of commaunding, but also of facultie & execution. This place then

E

beareth the spirits among the instruments; and as the soule is one, and indued with one only facultie, so the spirit is also one, and embraceth that one faculty, and distributeth it among the corporall members, as euerie one according to his diuerse temper or frame, or both ioyntly together is meete this way or that way to be employed; yet so that by degrees, and diuerse dispensations, it is communicated from the principall and chiefe partes with the rest. As first life and vitall spirit, from the hart to the rest by arteries: nourishment and growth, from the liuer by vaines: sense and motion, from the brayne by nerues: not confusedly, and by equall portions administred to all alike, but by such geometrical proportion as iustice requireth, and is necessary for the office of euerie part. Thus you see what nature the spirit is of, and to what vse it serueth in our nature, and of what sort of instrument it is to be accompted. The corporall part and mēbers, because their seruices be many are distinct into diuersitie of shapes and tempers, to answer all turnes; wherof some be more generall, and beare as it were office ouer the rest; as the heart is most generall, and extendeth it selfe to all the parts, with this prerogatiue aboue the liuer: that a part may liue for a time, and not be nourished, nether yet cā any part be nourished without life. This rule it exerciseth by the ministery of his arteries extended in branches throughout the bodie, and scattering the spirit of life throughout. Next the hart in vse and office towardes other members, the liuer obtaineth the second place:

by

by whose vertue, through the operation of the soule, and that spirituall hand, nourishment, and preparation of aliment is perfourmed in all the parts, vpon whom attendeth the stomach & the rest of the entralls vnder the midriffe. The third place is allotted to the braine, which by his sense and motion guideth, and directeth the partes maintained with life and nourishment: his sense is of two sorts, and so his motion, both inward, & outward. The inward sense, thinketh, imagineth and remembreth, and is practised with that peculiar temper and frame which the braine hath proper, as also his internall motion not much vnlike the panting of the hart. The outward sense and motion of sinewes is deriued from it into all parts that require sense, or mouing. The other partes subiect to these three principall and their ministers serue their owne turnes only, and are of priuate condition; except the soule command a voluntarie or mixed action: as to walke, to go &c. or to take breath, giue passage of stoole, or vrine.

CHAP. XIII.
How the soule by one simple facultie performeth so many and diuerse actions.

THvs haue you these partes, and organicall vses distinct: and if it seeme yet difficult vnto you, to conceaue, how one simple faculty can discharge such multiplicitie of actions, way with me a litle, by a comparison of similitude, the truth of this point, & accordingly accept it. We see it euident in automaticall instrumentes, as clockes, watches, and larums, howe one right and straight motion, through the aptnesse of the first wheele, not only causeth circular motion in the same, but in diuerse others also: and not only so, but distinct in pace, and time of motion: some wheeles passing swifter then other some, by diuerse rates: nowe to these deuises, some other instrument added, as hammer, and bell, not only another right motion springeth therof, as the stroke of the hammer, but sound also oft repeated, and deliuered it at certaine times by equall pauses; and that either larume or houres according as the partes of the clocke are framed. To these if yet moreouer a directorie hand be added; this first, and simple, and right motion by weight or straine, shall seeme not only to be author of deliberate sound, & to counterfet voyce, but also to point with the finger as much as it hath declared by sound. Besides these we see yet a third motion with reciprocation in the ballāce of the clocke. So many actions diuerse in kinde rise from one simple first motion, by reason of variety of ioynts in one engine. If to these you adde what wit can deuise, you may finde all the motion of heauen with his planets counterfetted, in a small modill, with distinction of time & season, as in the course of the heauenly bodies. And this appeareth in such sorte as carie their motion within them*selues. In water workes I haue seene a mill driuen with the winde, which hath both serued for grist, and auoyding of riuers of water out of drowned fennes and marishes; which to an American ignorant of the deuise, uife, would seeme to be wrought by a liuely actiō of euery part, and not by such a generall mouer as the wind is, which bloweth direct, & foloweth not by circular motion of the mill saile. Nowe if this be brought to passe in artificiall practises, & the varietie of action inferre not so many faculties, but meere dispositions of the instrumentes: let the similitude serue to illustrat that vnto you, whereto the reasons before alleaged, may with more force of proofe induce you. If yet you be not satisfied, (for melancholicke persons are for the most part doubtfull and least assured) and although ye acknowledge the truth hereof in organicall actions: yet in such as require no instrument, iudge otherwise; that scruple also by a similitude, I will take away and make it plaine vnto you, referring you for strength of reason to that which hath bene aforsayd. Before, I shewed the varietie of action, to spring of diuersitie of instrument; now, where there is no instrument, what diuersitie (say you) can there be? & yet to giue but one action to the soule, were to depriue it of many goodly exercises, whereby it apprehendeth the creator, thankfully acknowledgeth his goodnesse, and directeth it selfe to his honour, besides those spirituall offices, which the soules departed out of this life, in loue performe to ech other, with that knowledge of eternall things? It you require reason of proofe, the simplicitie of the soule, and the nature of diuerse things will make aunswer: if of illustration and comparison of similitude: then consider, howe with one viewe, a man beholdeth both top, and bottome of height, and both endes of length at once, the situation of the thing being conueniēt thereunto; yet are there neither diuerse faculties, nor diuerse inſtruments: the Sunne both ripeneth and withereth, and with an influence it bringeth forth mettals, trees, herbes, & whatſoeuer ſpringeth from the earth; ſome things it ſofteneth, and other ſome it hardeneth: other ſome it maketh ſweete, and other ſome bitter: an hammer driueth in, and driueth out, it looſeneth & faſteneth, it maketh & it marreth, not with diuerſity of faculty, keping the ſame waight temper, and faſhion it had before, but onely diuerſly applied, and vſed vpon diuerſe matters: ſo many vſes ariſe of one inſtrument. Moreouer, if a man were double fróted (as the Poets haue fained Ianus) & the inſtruments diſpoſed thereafter, the ſame facultie of ſight would addreſſe it ſelfe to ſee both before and behind at one inſtant, which nowe it doth by turning. As theſe actions of ſo ſundry ſorts require no diuerſe facultie, but chaunge of ſubiect, and altered application: ſo the mind, in action wonderfull, and next vnto the ſupreme maieſtie of God, and by a peculiar maner proceeding from him ſelfe, as the things are, ſubiect vnto the apprehenſion, & action thereof: ſo the ſame facultie varieth not by nature, but by vſe only, or diuerſity of thoſe thinges whereto it applieth it ſelfe: as the ſame facultie applied to differring things, diſcerneth: to thinges paſt, remembreth: to thinges future, foreſeeth: of preſent things determineth: and that which the eye doth by turning of the head,

beholding

Of Melancholie.

beholding before, behind, and on ech side, that doth the mind freely at once (not being hindered, nor reſtrained by corporall inſtrument) in iudging, remembring, foreſeeing, according as the thinges preſent them ſelues vnto the conſideration therof. For place mo then one, & where will you ſtay, and how will you number them? & why are there not as well three ſcore, as three? If you meaſure them by kindes of actions, they are indefinite, and almoſt infinite, and can not beare any certaine rate in our natures: ſeeing ſuch as are voluntarie, riſe vpon occaſions, and neceſſitie vncertaine: and naturall are diuerſe in euery ſeuerall part, and ſo according to their number are multiplied, and of them ſundrie actions being performed, as to attract, to concoct, to retaine, to expell, to aſſimilate, agglutinate, &c. not generally, but the peculiar and proper nouriſhment, the number would fill vp Eraſtoſthenes ſiue to count thē all. Wherfore to conclude this argument, and to leaue you reſolued in this point, let the facultie be one, and pluralitie in applicatiō, vſe, & diuerſitie of thoſe things whereabout it was conuerſaunt: otherwiſe the mind ſhalbe diſtracted into parts, which is whole in euery part: and admit mixture, which is moſt ſimple: and become ſubiect of diuerſe qualities, which are diſtinct in nature, and communicated by mixture of ſubſtances whereto they belong, & not confuſed together in one, againſt nature. Thus you haue mine opinion touchinge theſe three parts: of ſoule, of ſpirit, and bodie, with their peculiar actions, and howe euerie one is

E iiij

seuerally brought to passe: which I thought necessary first to make plaine, before I entred into particular aunswer to the former obiections, as the grounde of the solution, and rule whereto the particular aunswers are to be squared. So then I take generally the soule to be affected of the bodie and spirit, as the instrument hindreth the worke of the artificer; which is not by altering his skill, or diminishing his cunning, but by deprauing the action through vntowardnesse of toole, and fault of instrument. This in the Chapter following, I will particularly apply to the former obiections.

Chap. XIIII.
The particular aunswere to the obiections made in the 11 Chapter.

AS for those faculties which age seemeth not only to alter, but also to breede, they are altogether organicall, and are not of this or that sorte: or appeare not, because, the faculty suffereth violence or wanteth, but because the instrumentes as yet lacked such disposition, as the soule requireth, being altogether vnapt, or else although faulty in parte, yet employed as they may be: whereupon the actions become imperfect. As the brayne in a child new borne, ouercharged with humidity causeth discretiõ of sensible obiectes for 40 dayes, as sayeth Hippocrates and Aristotle, to be so dull, that they feele not, though they be rubbed, neither laugh they, though they be tickled, as afterward they doe both

Of Melancholie. 73

both, and take pleasure in the one, and as we be
affected after a mixt sorte in the other: which
obscurity of sence, ioyned with want of experience of sensible thinges, and comparing of their
euents, with want of exercise, is the cheefe cause
of that simplicity of children in affaires of this
life, wherein prudence is most conuersant. For
better conceiuing of which point, you are to vnderstand, or call to minde, how the soule hath
certaine principles of knowledge ingenerate,
called Criteria of the Greekes, and certaine taken from obseruation of sensible thinges, and
from them framed, agreeably to those grounded
principles and ingenerate knowledge of the
soule. These Criteria discerne betwixt good and
badde, trueth and falshood, and are euer firme,
and certayne in themselues, and are abused only by the imperfection of such instrumentes, by
which the discretion and report of outward obiectes do passe. From this do springe three seuerall actions, whereby the whole course of reason
is made perfect. First, that which the greekes cal
Sinteresis, the ground, whereupon the practise
of reason consisteth, aunswering the proposition
in a sillogisme: the conscience applying, the assumption: and of them both, the third, a certaine
trueth concluded: these partes the soule doth
without instrument of body, and neuer faileth
therein, so farre as the naturall principles lead,
or outward obiectes be sincerely taken, & truely
reported to the minds consideration. From the
practises of these ingenerate, & infallible grouds
rise all the knowledge of outward thinges, and

humane sciences: and as a rule being but one ruleth equally gold, timber, and stone, and the ballance peaseth all kinde of waighty things alike, so these applied to practises of life, & wordly busines, haue ingendred prudence, and circumspection: in the conuersation of men, and maner of behauiour, the morall vertues: In the perfection of voluntary actions, diuerse artes and sciences, and aboue all, disposeth it selfe to the worship and adoration of God, in some one sort or other: the right manner whereof depending vpon his expresse oracles, and operation of his spirite aboue nature: the want wherof hath caused so many rites, and sundry superstitiós as are, and haue bene accompted religion in the world, the humaine sense being neither able to deliuer misteries of such diuine quality vnto the minde, and those groundes and rules being feebled, and crooked in that kinde, by the degenerate state of our first parentes. So then that wherein children seeme to fayle through age in reason, is not that the faculty is vnripe, or to seeke: but because the exercise thereof through necessity of life, is employed in such thinges, as sense not being before acquainted with, maketh offer therof to the mindes iudgement confused, and deliuereth one thing for another, or the same not sincerely: so the fault is in organicall action, and not in ingenerate faculty, which organe hath not yet, the full disposition of all his partes, or mistaketh for want of experience, that which it reporteth: according to which the minde pronounceth, directed by her ingenerate science:

which

which both are manifest in tender yeares: whose braines are so soked, and drowned with naturall moisture, that in them the animall instrumentes are most feeble, especially such as require vse of the braine it selfe the moistest part of all the body, the other actions which stand of a passiue disposition (as outward sense) being litle or nothing thereby hindered. This appeareth plainly in those things which children do distinctly cōprehend, which their ingenerate science, essentiall to the minde, doth clearely, and perfectly conceiue and iudge, as the auncient: as a child knowing the heate of fire, will as readely iudge of the perrill, as the wisest Senatour, of the inroad of a borderer, or the politick captaine, of the vnequall encoūter with his enimy, by place, occasion, of time, or what opportunity so euer, & hauing felt the heat thereof, will as presently iudge the sentence false, affirmeth it could, as the sharpest witted philosopher, the most captious argumēt, & subtilest Sorites of Stilpo. Moreouer we dayly see in children a Preludium as it were, & draught of the grauest actions, that in earnest do afterward fall out in our life, only the thing altered wherin the minde is occupied. For they will both counterfet the wise counseller, & the valiant captaine: the Maiesty of a prince, & duety of homage and subiection, and giue signification for the most part of that hope in their youth, as a modill, wherof age afterward maketh full proofe: which as it appeareth in all, so most notably in the worthy Cyrus, of whose education Zenophon writeth. Now it also appeareth in children (as their organicall partes are tempered,) more quickely, to apprehend, euē thofe childifh matters wherewith they bufie thēfelues or they therewith more or leffe acquainted: which both concurred in Cyrus: his body being as it fhould feeme of excellent temper, and himfelfe, fonne of a King, at thofe dayes the great maifter of the world: as for his education, it was nothing elfe, but an acquainting of his minde with thofe excellent partes of a prince, which afterward being at full hability of inftrument, he put in practife, as his gouernment required. This called Plato a remembrance only, and calling to minde againe of thofe thinges, which the foule, by being plunged in this gulfe of the body, had forgotten: which I fo farre otherwife count of as neither do I hold that the foule had euer before any knowledge of thefe outward thinges, and fuch whereof the fenfes be motions, neither being feparated from this corporall fociety, fhall haue any knowledge, or remembrance of hereafter, at leaft in this maner, but only is conuerfant in thofe exercifes which require no bodely organ, till the refurrection, when ioyned to the body againe, as after a fleepe, it recondeth with frefh memory what it hath done good or euill, with confcience excufing or accufing: becaufe they rife of fenfe, and fenfible obiectes, and haue no farther vfe then in humane fociety, which fuch actions do vphold: neither carieth it away more then it brought, as whereto nothing can be added. That then, which generally I aunfwered, touching organical practifes peculiar to bodie

OF MELANCHOLIE.

dy and spirite, the same doe I apply particularly to the obiection from age, and such discretion as it bringeth with it; euen that all such are actions depending vpon instrument, wherunto the faule whatsoeuer is to be ascribed, and not vnto any faculty of the minde, (which neuer suffereth increase nor decrease, or any other kinde of alteration,) or else vnto want of experience, & exercise of those things, which greater yeares medle with: wherein the senses both externall, and internall by vse being perfect, like as a true looking glasse representeth the countenance to the eye, in all pointes as nature, hath framed it, so offer they the relation true & distinct from sensible thinges: whereof the minde deliuereth resolution and sentence: willeth good thinges, and refuseth the contrarie, whatsoeuer it seemeth to do otherwise, through the inordinate instrumēts the seates of vnruly appetite, and disorderly affection, far different from that which the minde it selfe willeth entirely, free from all perturbation. That which I haue answered concerning the animall actions, fitteth also the obiection of propagation: for such partes haue not as yet their naturall disposition thereunto: neither doth the animall partes make such discretion in male and female, whereof that appetite ariseth, although the sight and countenance and person of eche party be all one: neither is any faculty idle at any time, (the instruments only of sense and motion take refreshing by rest,) especially so many yeares: which must needes ensue, if it were a faculty distinct, and not rather according to the aptnes of inftrument, a peculiar exercife only. For nature employeth all to the vttermoft, and giueth neuer ouer, except it be more chearefully and ftrongly to lay hand to the worke againe, which to propagation needeth not, no vfe hauing bene thereof at all before. If you fay it rifeth of an internall conceite, take this withall, that the conceite is taken from an external obiect, together with a difpofed parte thereunto, which fo foone as it is perfected to the vfe: the minde being alwayes occupied, and in continuall motion, employeth that alfo whereunto naturally it is bent. The obiection rifing from cuftome of life in faylers, butchers, and ploughmé, receiueth the fame anfwere. For their inftruments of action through continuall practife of fuch artes, maketh them in common fenfe, imagination, and affection, to deliuer thinges vnto the minde after an impure fort, alwayes fauouring of their ordinary trade of life. This is that putteth of butchers from iuries, and iudgeméts of life and death amongeft men: who although they know there is difference betwixt man and beaft, the caufe of the one and the vfe of the other, the giltles prifoner, and the innocent lamb, yet they being accuftomed with flaughter, the difference is not fo fincerely taken, and the affection not indifferent in fuch a cafe: and therefore from fuch capitall caufes they are remoued. The mariner as the Europians are more rough, bold, hardie, inconftant, thé the Afians, through inconftancy of the aire, and tempeftioufnes of the regions: fo the incertainty of the weather,

and

and stormie seas with custome of daunger, maketh them more rough, bold, and hastie, then they which be of other trade of life, and their businesse on firme land: euery action in respect and comparison of due consideration, is either winde, tide, or tépest; the ancher, saile, or steirne: euery displeasure a storme, and euery contentment a calme: euen as a man that hath trauelled all the day on horsebacke, or sailed on the sea, though he be laid on his bed, yet keepeth an imagination of trauell still, his body fairing after a sort, as though it were on horsebacke, or yet embarked, iudgeth not so lightly of rest: by reason of the former inured trauell: so these men through their kind of life, either by false representatiós of such obiects, or imperfect & mixed report, offer things to the mind, otherwise then they are indeed, and receiue iudgement of them thereafter: whereto their affections answering, they take things in farre other part, then they shold, or the nature of the cause requireth: Now the region or habitation being as it were aparant vnto vs, ministring breath and foode, no maruell if our bodies be affected thereafter, & so the actions varie (as the child of the parentes in one sort or other carieth the resemblaunce) the facultie being all one, and keeping the same state, while the instrumets stand to such hazard, as outward thinges, either by region, diet, custome of life, or else whatsoeuer doth threaten and bring vpon vs. Most of all hath region this force, not onely in that we feede as the soyle affordeth, but because the aire whereof the spirits of our bodies are repaired, besides that which riseth of the internall spirit of aliment, is continually drunke in vs, and passeth into all the secrets of our intrailes, stirreth our humours, and diuersly affecteth all our organical partes: as the aire and soile, drie, open, & barren, maketh the bodies firme, hard, and compact, and the spirits pure & subtile, wherby what action soeuer is to be performed of them, is more quicke, nimble, and prompt, especially it nourishmet be proportionall, then of people of contrary habitation. Of all the former obiections, the humors of our bodies seeme most to vrge, & chalenge interest in disposing of the mind, both in respect of those accidents, we see persons fall into ouercharged with them, as also, because commonly the affections of the hart, as ioy, sadnesse, delight, displeasure, hope, feare, or whatsoeuer else of them is mixed among the perturbations, commonly are all to them ascribed, which because it most concerneth the chiefe drift of this discourse of melancholy, I will more stand vpon, and afford it a more copious answer.

Chap. XV.
Whether the perturbations rise of the humour or not.

THE perturbations are taken commonlie to rise of melancholy, choler, bloud, or fleume; so that men of hastie disposition we call cholericke: of sad, melancholicke: of heauie and dull flegmaticke: of merie and chearfull, sanguine:

and

OF MELANCHOLIE.

and not onely the common opinion so taketh it but these affections are accompted of the Phisitians for tokens of such cōplexions, & such humours raigning in the bodie. Let vs consider therfore, whether the truth be as they hold it, & perturbations haue no other fountaine thē these humours. What these humours are, we haue sufficiently declared, and how they are ingendred: the vse of them is to nourish the parts of the bodie, and to repaire the continuall expence therof through trauelles of this life; besides that, which the naturall heat continually consumeth. The perturbations thus moue vs, disturbe our counsels, & disquiet our bodies on this sort. First occasion riseth from outward things, wherin we either take pleasure, or wherewith we are offended: this obiect is caried to the internall senses from the outward; which if it be a matter sensuall onely, the minde vseth to impart it to the hart, by the organicall internall senses, which with ioy embraceth it, or with indignation, and mislike refuseth it; if of such points, as it selfe liketh, without their helpe it giueth knowledge thereof to the hart by the spirits, which either embraceth the same, impelled by the minds willing, or reiecteth it with mislike and hatred, according to her nilling. But before I proceed further in this Chapter, it shall be necessarie to declare vnto you, all the sortes of perturbations, which being distinguished vnto classes or proper families, shall deliuer great light vnto vs: both in laying open their natures, and also compared with the nature of the humours, make

F

more cleare demonstration, what likelihoode they carie to be effects of such causes as the humours are. All perturbations are either simple, or cōpounded of the simple. Simple are such, as haue no mixture of any other perturbation: and these are either primitiue, and first, or deriuatiue and drawne from them. The primitiues haue like or dislike properties vnto thē. Loue & hate are the first kinds and primitiues of the rest: loue being a vehement liking, and hate a vehement affection of disliking: from these springe all the deriuatiues, which arise either from loue, or hate, like, or dislike. From loue and liking of a present good, springeth ioy and reioycing; if it be to come, hope entertaineth the hart with expectation. From dislike and hate: if the thing be euill as the other good, (in deede or in apparance it skilleth not) and present, riseth heauinesse of hart, and disposition of sadnesse: if it be a future euill, feare riseth frō the mislike of hate; & these I take to be all the simple perturbations. The compound, are such as haue part of the simple by mixture: and that either of the primitiue simple, or the deriuatiue: and of the primitiues with simple ones only, or mixed with deriuatiues. Such are mixed with primitiues onely, are either mixed vnequally, of loue and liking, or of mislike & hate; or equally of thē both. Of the first sort, & taking more part of liking, is the affection which moueth vs to laugh; thus we cal merinesse wherwith we with some discontentment, take pleasure at that, which is done or sayd ridiculously: of which sort are deeds, or wordes, vnseemely or vnmeet, and yet moue no compassiō;

as when a man scaldeth his mouth with his pottage or an hote pie, we are discōtented with the hurt, yet ioye at the euent vnexpected of the partie, and that we haue escaped it; frō whence commeth laughter: which because it exceedeth the mislike of the thing that hurteth, bursteth out into vehemency on that side, and procureth that merie gesture. If on the other side the thing be such as the mislike excedeth the ioy we haue of our freedome from that euill, then riseth pity and compassion: and these perturbations take their beginninges of the primitiues vnequally mixed, whereby one of them doth after a sorte obscure the other. The other are such as haue equall mixture, and those are enuie and iclosie. If the thing we loue be such as we haue not part of, then springeth an hate or mislike of the partie who enioyeth that we want and like of, and so breedeth enuy, a griefe for the prosperity of another, or good successe whatsoeuer, wherein we haue no part. If it be such benefit as we enioy, and are grieued it should be communicated with other, and wherein we refuse a pattener, that is called iclousie: and is seene manifest in such, as ar amorously affected, or of a'piring natures: and these are compounded of the primitiues alone, like or mislike, loue, or hate. Those which are mixed of primitiues, or deriuatiues, are of two sortes, according as the primitiues: that is to say mixed of loue or hate. Nowe loue mixed with hope, breedeth trust: with loue and feare distrust. Hate or mislike compounded with hope, breedeth anger: whereby we are displeased with that misliketh vs , and by hope of being satisfied of that, that offered the dislike, are driuen to anger the affection of reuenge. If it be any thing wherein we haue displeased our selues with, it is called shame : if it be compounded with feare, it is called bashfulnesse; if the mislike be taken from another, the composition is of hate and anger, and thereof springeth, malice. Thus haue you the perturbations compounded of primitiue passions with their deriuatiues. Of deriuatiues betwixt them selues arise dispaire, and confident assurance. Dispaire is compounded of heauinesse, griefe and feare: the other of ioy and hope: thus haue you after my minde the perturbations raunged into their seuerall classes: to the ende,the affinitie of cause and effect (if any be) betwixt them and the humours, may more easily appeare; if none be, as in deed there is none,then the contrarie truth may with greater euidence , approue it selfe vnto your iudgement. For loue or liking, hate or mislike, being but two primitiue passions, howe may we with reason referre them to the humours,which are foure: and if the perturbations should rise of humour, then should they aunswer ech other neither mo nor fewer : and as the one is compound, primitiue and deriuatiue, so should the humours be at the instant of those passions, which is impossible: or if they be not at the instant mixed, but before , the hart should not lye indifferent to all passions,and the mixture being once made , by what meanes should they be againe vnmixed? Againe if they rise of humour,

then

then should those parts wherein humours most abound, be instruments of passions, and so the gall of anger, and the splene of sadnesse, and not the hart, which is the seate of all those affectiõs, which we call perturbations: from which both of those partes, are parted by the midriffe. But you will say: these affections rise of the temper of the hart, and that temper of the humour. Not so: for either the affections rise of the frame alone of the hart, or else at the least ioyned with the temper: nowe the humours haue so small force in making temper, and framing the complexion, that them selues are all therof framed, the spirits applying the temper of the organical parts to that businesse. Touching the frame of the hart, such as haue bin most couragious haue it of substance firme, compact, and of qualitie moderate, the poores neither ouerlarge nor narowe: in which points the temper and complexion hath no vse: but the frame alone. Againe, these passions being wrought of the heart by a certaine enlarging of it selfe, if it be pleased, and closing, if it be contrarily affected: which be actions not of complexion, but of frame & shape, make sufficient proofe against the complexion in this parte, which only beareth it self affected to that which it toucheth, altering it, if it be of victualls into humours, and the humours into the substance of the body, which it indueth with the same complexion. Againe it fareth oft times that this or that humour aboundeth by disordered diet, yet the complexion all one; neither purgations of humour alter complexion, a fixed thing, ingenerate by nature, & not ouerthrown but by some venimous qualitie direct opposit against it, or long custome of other disorder, whereby nature is supplanted in time, & growing in acquaintāce, with which first is misliked, is ouermatched with a counterfet nature, gotten by vse of that otherwise is vnnaturall. These points might be more at large layed open, if it were necessarie, or they did not withdraw from the purpose I haue in hand, to rest more vppon them. But how then cometh it to passe, that melancholicke persons are more sad then other, & cholericke more angrie &c. if these humoures beare no sway herein? For answer of which question, you are to vnderstand that both ioye and sadnesse are of two sorts, as also the rest springing from them: the one is naturall rising vpon an outward accasion, if the bodie be well tempered, and faultles in his instruments, and the obiect made no greater nor lesse then it is in deed, and the hart, aunswer proportionally therunto: the other is vnnaturall, and disordered, rising either of no outward occasion, but from inward delusion, or else such as are (by fault of the report of the senses, or euil disposition of the hart) otherwise taken then the obiect requireth. In this second kind, the humours seeme to haue greatest rule, which whether they haue so, as causes or not, & in what respect they entermeddle, I wil now make plaine vnto you. Of the first sort of perturbations naturall, and rising vppon euident occasion I neede stand lesse vpon, seing as the hart is by outward causes moued, so is it

neither

neither more affected of this humour then of that, neither can there be any such sudden separation of humours be wrought in the bodie, whereby through anger choler should disioyne him selfe from his fellow humours, and possesse the hart: or melancholie in causes of griefe, sorowe, or feare, especially an humour of grosse & earthy partes, as it were the very lies of the rest of the bloud. Againe, it were verie contrarie to reason, to attribute an action of so necessary vse, as are the perturbations vnto that, which is no organe of our bodies, but only matter of foode and nourishment; of which sort are all the humours, keeping them selues within compasse of good temper. Moreouer if through anger the hart be moued first, then is it first troubled, and the perturbations wrought, before the humour receaue impression: if the humor admit first the motion of the thing louely or hurtfull, & impart that to the heart, then should it receiue a degree of excellencie aboue the hart in this respect, being more attendant vpon the spirit, the chiefe steward of this facultie, then the hart is, which next to the spirit hath greatest place in the bodie. But why thē say you, haue the Philosophers defined anger a boyling of the bloud about the hart? if it be according to that definition, then the more cholericke a man is, so much the more angry is he: because the choler is first apt to boyle, as it were brimstone to the match, in respect of the other humours. That definition of anger, is to be taken not by proper speech, but by a metonymicall phrase, whereby the cause is

F iiij

attributed to the effect. For first the heart moueth, kindled with anger, then the bloud riseth, which being cholericke encreaseth the heate, but addeth nothing to the passion: nowe because we sensibly feele an extraordinarie heate about our hearts when we be moued to angrie passions, therefore they haue defined anger by that effect: which boyling, riseth not of the quality of the bloud, but by a strife of a contrary motion in the heart at one time, the one being a contraction of it selfe, and a retraite of the bloud and certaine spirits not farre of: with mislike of that offendeth, as in feare, which commandeth euen from the extreme and vtmost parts: whereby it gathereth great heate within, which breathing out againe with reuenge, causeth through vehemency, & suddennesse of the motion, that boyling of heat, procured of anger: especially if it be not deliuered by word and deede, whereby liberty is giuen for the passion to breake foorth, which restrained in any sort, breedeth an agony of such feruency, as it may resemble the scalding of a boyling chaldron not vncouered, or an hote furnace closed vp in all vents. Moreouer if perturbation should be caused of humour, to whether should we attribute it? to the naturall humor, or to the excrement? the excrement is far remoued frō the hart, & is not so ready to affect it, a great distāce being betwixt their seuerall places; & in iaūdes, the gal ouerflowing the body, & passing through the vaines, & staining all parts, we see them not so affected, more angry then at other times, or their bodies being cleered from the

the tincture of yellownes. If it be the naturall humor, that is to say, the subtilest part of the bloud, alwayes contained in the hart (whether you vnderstand that bloud which is comprehended in the two bosoms, or that wherwith the hart is sustained & nourished in euery part) why is not thē the hart alwayes affected without intermission, with such passions as the bloud enclineth vnto, seeing it is alwayes present, & keepeth his disposition alike? If you will haue it of neither, but of that which is cōtained in the great vain, rushing with violence into the right side of the hart, the quality of that bloud being of cooler temper thē that which the heart hath already embraced, should serue to mitigate the mood, rather then to adde mo stickes to the fire. To conclude this point, lest I should seeme to fight with a shadow: if either humor, or excrement should haue part in mouing affections, no counsel of philosophy, nor precept of wise men were comparable to calme these raging passions, vnto the purging potions of Phisitians, & in this case the Elleborans of Anticera; the Colocynthis of Spaine, and the Rhubarb of Alexādria, aboue all the schools of Diuinitie or Philosophy. The lesse I labour against these humors in the kinds of naturall perturbations, or such as rise vpon occasion, because I thinke the errour is sone remoued, & requireth no long reasoning. The other sort which moue vs without cause, or externall obiect, either to sadnes, anger, feare, or ioy, because they seeme altogither to be effects of humors, no other cause being apparent whereto to ascribe them, I will more copiously debate this point in the Chapter following.

Chap. XVI.

VVhether perturbatiōs, which are not moued by outward occasions rise of humours or not: and how?

WE do see by experience certaine persons which enioy all the comfortes of this life whatsoeuer wealth can procure, and whatsoeuer friendship offereth of kindnes, and whatsoeuer security may assure them: yet to be ouerwhelmed with heauines, and dismaide with such feare, as they can neither receiue consolation, nor hope of assurance, notwithstanding ther be neither matter of feare, or discontentment, nor yet cause of daunger, but contrarily of great cōfort, and gratulation. This passiō being not moued by any aduersity present or imminent, is attributed to melancholie the grossest part of all the blood, either while it is yet contained in the vaines: or aboundeth in the splene, (ordained to purge the blood of that drosse and setling of the humours) surcharged therwith for want of free uent, by reason of obstruction, or any wayes else the passage being let of cleare auoydance. The rather it seemeth to be no lesse, because purgation, opening of a vayne, diet, and other order of cure and medicine, as phisick prescribeth, haue bene meanes of chaunging this disposition, and mitigatiō of those sorowes, and quieting of such feares, as melancholie persons haue fancied to themselues, & haue as it seemeth restored both wit and courage. Hitherto we haue bene led by reason of the obiection from humors, which imported

ported great power in them of affecting the minde. It was anſwered before generally, whatſoeuer was done in the body of any parte to be done organically, and that was applied ſpecially to certaine obiections before aunſwered: it remaineth here, that the ſame be applyed alſo to our humours, which haue no other power to affect the minde, then to alter the ſtate of the inſtrumentes: which next to the minde, & ſoule it ſelfe are the only cauſes of all direct action in the body. So here we are to conſider, in what ſort the humours moue theſe perturbations aboue mentioned: whether as cheefe workers, inſtruments, or other kinde of helpers: and ſo how they may claime any intereſt in terrifying, or ſoliciting the minde, this way or that way, as the obiections before mentioned would beare vs in hand. It hath ben declared before how the mind is the ſole mouer in the body, and how the reſt of the partes fare as inſtrumentes, and miniſters: whereby in naturall affections the humors are ſecluded from cheefe doers, and being no organicall partes ſerue for no inſtrumentes. For whatſoeuer hath any conſtant and firme action in our bodies, the ſtate of health remayning firme, is done either by ſoule, or by the partes of the body: of which the humours are neither, and ſo vtterly ſecluded of nature from any peculiar actiõ to any vſe of the body. For that they are ſaid to nouriſh, it ſignifieth only a paſſiue diſpoſition, by which through our nouriſhing power, they receiue the Character of our nature, and are altered into the ſubſtance of the same, they themselues giuing ouer their priuate actiō, and submitting to the naturall concoctiue vertue, which destroyeth all particularities of nourishment, and bringeth them to that vniformity which our nature requireth. Then while the body is in health, the humors beare no sway of priuate action, but it being once altered, and they euill disposed, and breaking from that regiment whereunto they should be subiect, are so farre off from subiection to the disposition of our bodies, and strength of our partes, that they oppresse them, and as it appeareth in simptomaticall euentes in sicknes, dispise that gouernment, wherto by natures law they stand bound. Thus then I hold humours to be occasions of disorderly perturbations, euen as they are meanes of deprauing the instrument of perturbation, and turning it otherwise, then nature hath disposed, whose gouernment when it hath shaken of, it affecteth vs two maner of wayes: the one by the corporall substance, whereby it annoyeth the corporall masse of bodies, and complexion, and breaketh out into soares, Emposthumes, or other such anoyances: the other by a spirit which it possesseth, either contrary altogether, or diuerse at the least from ours, wherewith many wayes it disturbeth the orderly actions, & weakneth the vigor of the same: now both by substance, and by spirite it altereth complexion where it preuaileth, and thereby giueth greatest stroake to the organicall members. Then seing all actions are performed both by spirite and corporall instrument, and the humours exceeding

OF MELANCHOLIE.

ding the gouernment of nature, and withdrawing themselues from subiection thereof, affect vs both wayes, spirite against spirite, and corporall substance against his like, we are to cōsider, how by these two meanes our actions suffer through their disorder, and where their operation taketh most place in working such phantasticall perturbations wherewith we are deluded. Of all partes of the body, in ech perturbation, two are cheifly affected: first the brayne, that both apprehendeth the offensiue or pleasaunt obiect, & iudgeth of the same in like sort, and communicateth it with the harte, which is the second part affected: these being troubled carie with them all the rest of the partes into a simpathy, they of all the rest being in respect of affection of most importance. The humours then to worke these effectes, which approch nigh to naturall perturbations grounded vpon iust occasion, of necessity, alter either brayne or hart: if the brayne be altered, and the obiect not rightly apprehended then is it deliuered otherwise then it standeth in nature, and so the hart moued to a disorderly passion. Againe though the brayne be without faulte, and report delyuered to the hart sincerely: yet that being distempered, or altered in cōplexion by faulte of humour, doth not aunswere in affection as the obiect requireth: but more or lesse, as the distemper misleadeth: if both partes be ouercharged of humour, the apprehension & affection both are corrupted, and misse of their right action, and so all thinges mistaken, ingender that confused spirite, and those stormes of

outragious loue, hatred, hope or feare, wherewith bodies so passionate are here and there, tossed with disquiet. Now particularly the spirite of the humour being subtiler, thinner, and hoter then is meete, maketh the apprehension quicker then it should be, and the discretion more hasty, then is meete for the vpright deliuery to the hart, what to embrace or to refuse: this causeth pronenes to anger, when we are offended without cause, commonly called teastines, and frowardnes. If the humour also with his spirite possesse the brayne, then are these passions of longer continuance: humour being of a more sollid nature then the spirite, and so not easily dispersed, which causeth fittes of such passiōs to be of longer continuance: and thus the hart may be abused from the brayne: not much vnlike as it falleth often out in communication of speach amongest vs: a man of hasty disposition, ready to aunswere, and quick witted, will make reply to that which should be said, before the tale be halfe told, whereby he faileth in his replication, and aunswereth from the purpose: which if he had bene first assured, wherto to reply, he should not haue missed. This appeareth plaine in Cholericke persons, or such as are disposed to anger: such are offended where they haue no cause in truth, but by mistaking: and where they haue cause the vehemency of the apprehension, and the suddénes of the report from the brayne vnto the seate of perturbation, inforceth double the passion: especially when the hart is as flexible, as the brayne is light: then raungeth it into all
extre-

extremity. This commeth to passe, not by any power of anger in the Cholerick humour: but by reason the instrumentes are misordered, either by vapour rising from that humour, or the very substance of the same. They are disordered in this sort through Choler. The naturall spirit and complexiō of these partes become subtiler, thinner, and quicker, proner to action, then of their natures they should be, through the heat which riseth of Choler, and his spirit intermixed with ours: by this mobility of vapour, our spirit (of a quieter and more stable disposition,) is either made more rare, then is expedient for the vse of our bodies, or else striuing as it were to subdue this bastard spirite and vnwelcome ghest, can not giue that attendance vpon his proper duety, which naturally it should: and so the actions thereupon rise depraued, and hauing wherwith it is encumbred within, admitteth the cause of displeasure more easily which riseth abroad: being an additiō to that which molesteth at home: and these natures for the most parte are troubled with a Cholerick humour, or fretting, like to Choler, about the mouth of the stomach, which is of all the inward partes of quickest sense and feeling. This causeth them, especially fasting, before the humour be mitigated, and delayed with nourishment, to be most prone to that angry passion. The teasty waywardnes of sick persons, such as are vexed with payne or feauer, wherby the humors of the body become more fell maketh euident proofe hereof. We see how small matters put them out of patience, &

euery thing offendeth: whereas in health the same occasions would litle, or nothing moue. The reason is because, they measure all outward accidents, by that they finde of discontentment within: not that the humor that discontenteth is any instrument of passion, or carieth with it faculty to be displeased: but because it disquieteth the body, and giueth discontentment to nature, it is occasion why displeasures are made great: and where there is no cause, nature troubled within, faireth as greatly displeased with that which outwardly should not displease: the griefe within, being added to an indifferēt thing without, and drawing it into like felowship of displeasure, euen but for that it pleaseth not: like as in a troubled sea, a great vessell is more easily stirred with smal strength, then in the calme hauen, or quiet streame: so our spirites, and organicall instruments of passion, the parte tossed with stormy weather of internall discontentment, is with litle occasion disquieted, yea with the shaking of a rush, that hath no show of calming those domesticall stormes, that arise more troublesome, and boisterous to our nature, then all the blustering windes in the Ocean, sea. For when our passion is once vp by such occasion, the commō sense is also caried therewith, and distinction of outward thinges hindered at the least, if not taken away, all things being wayed by that which nature findeth offēce at within: euen as the tast altered in feauers by cholerick vapours, maketh sweete thinges seeme bitter, and vnpleasaunt, which of themselues are most delectable to the taste,

OF MELANCHOLIE.

tast, and would greatly satisfie the same partie, the bitter relish through that taint of choller once taken away. And in this sort in my opinion ariseth the disorderly, & vnruly passion of choller, both increased, where some occasion is offered, and procured by inward disposition of the bodie and spirit, when there is no pretence, or shewe of cause. This is seene as plainly in mirth and ioye, which riseth as well vpon inward harmonie of spirit, humour, and complexion, as vpon glad tidings, or externall benefite whereof we take reioycing. A bodie of sanguine complexion (as commonly we call it, although complexion be another thing, then condition of humors) the spirits being in their iust temper in respect of qualitie, and of such plenty as nature requireth, not mixed or defiled, by any straunge spirit or vapor, the humours in quantity & qualitie rated in geometricall, and iust proportion, the substance also of the bodie, and all the members so qualified by mixture of elementes, as all conspire together in due proportion, breedeth an indifferencie to all passions. Nowe if bloud abound, and keepe his sincerity, and the body receaue by it, and the spirits rising from the same, a comfort in the sensible partes, without doubt then, as anger without cause externall, rose vpō inward displeasure; so this spirit, these humours, and this temper, may moue an inward ioy, wherof no externall obiect may be accompted as iust occasion. This is the cause that maketh some men prone to ioy, and laughter at such thinges, as other men are not drawne with into any pas-

G

sion, and maketh them picke out, and seeke for causes of laughter, not onely to moue others to the like, but to expresse their mery passiō, which riseth by the iudgement of our senses imparted to the hart, not regarding whether the cause be inward or outward, that moueth, which taketh comfort thereat, as though the obiect were externall. This especially commeth to passe if the bloud be such about the hart, as his purenesse & sincerenesse with sweetnesse that carieth moderation of temper doth so comfort, and mollifie it, that it easily, & aptly enlargeth it selfe thē such bloud or such vapor that hath this tickling qualitie, causeth a delight conceiued in the braine, and communicated with the hart, procureth a comfortable gratulation, and inward ioy of that whereof nature taketh pleasure. For as we haue sights, tastes, smelles, noyses, pleasant obiectes without vs, and on the contrary part, as manie odious, and hatefull, which do force our senses: so haue we also all these internall, pleasaunt or vnpleasaunt: & as we haue of sensuall obiects internall, so in like manner pleasure & displeasure is communicated frō within of the braine to the heart, of such things as we are not able directly to referre to this or that qualitie: as we see it fareth with tasts oftentimes: such mixtures may be in sauces, that something may please vs we cannot expresse what, raysed of the compositiō. This chiefly falleth to our bodies, when that which giueth this occasion carieth force of gentle and light spirits: as wine, and strong drinke, and all aromaticall spices, which haue a power

OF MELANCHOLIE. 99

to comfort the braine, and hart, and affect all our bodie throughout with celeritie and quickneſſe, before their ſpirits be ſpent in the paſſage: then the braine giueth merie report, & the hart glad for it ſelfe, and all the fellow members, as it were, daunceth for ioy, and good liking, which it receaueth of ſuch internall prouocations. Thē as we ſee wine giue occaſion of mirth by his excellent ſpirit, wherewith our ſpirit is delighted, and greatly increaſed, if it be drunke with moderation; ſo ſuch as are of merie diſpoſitions, enioy a naturall wine in their bodies, eſpecially harts & braines, which cauſeth them to laugh at the wagging of a feather, and without iuſt matter of laughter, without modeſt regard of circūſtance, to beare them ſelues light & ridiculous: & this my friende *M.* I take to be the cauſe of merrie greekes, who ſeeke rather to diſcharge them ſelues of the iocond affection, ſtirred vp by their humour, then require true outward occaſion of ſolace and recreation. Nowe as before I haue ſayd that choler procureth anger, not as cauſe, but as occaſion, ſo likewiſe bloud thus tempered and repleniſhed with theſe aromaticall and merie ſpirits, giueth occaſion only of this pleaſantneſſe, and is no cauſe thereof, the hart making iuſt claime to theſe affections as the only inſtrument, & vnder the ſoule, chiefe author of theſe vnruly companions: which inſtrument is ſo diſpoſed, that obeying the mind, and thoſe naturall rules whereby all things are eſteemed, good or bad, true or falſe, to be done or not to be done, no otherwiſe then by a ciuill ſubiection ruled by

G ij

counsell & no constraint, it repugneth oft times all the strong cōclusions whatsoeuer reason can make to the contrary. Thus you vnderstād how a man may be angrie and merie without externall obiect, or outward cause: now let vs consider, howe sadnesse and feare, the points which most belong to this discourse, and your present state, may also arise without occasion of outward terror either presently molesting, or fearing vs by likelihood, or possibility of future danger. As the nature of choler is subtile, hote, bitter, and of a fretting and biting qualitie, both it selfe and the vapors that passe from it, and bloud temperate, sweet, and full of cheerefull and comfortable spirits, answerable to those we haue ingenerate, especially if they become aromaticall, as I may terme them, and of a fragrant nature, by naturall temper, or by meanes of diet: so melancholie of qualitie, grosse, dull, and of fewe comfortable spirits; and plentifully replenished with such as darken all the clernesse of those sanguineous, and ingrosse their subtilnesse, defile their purenesse with the fogge of that slime, and fennie substance, and shut vp the hart as it were in a dungeon of obscurity, causeth manie fearefull fancies, by abusing the braine with vglie illusions, & locketh vp the gates of the hart, whereout the spirits should breake forth vpon iust occasion, to the comfort of all the family of their fellowe members: whereby we are in heauinesse, sit comfortlesse, feare, distrust, doubt, dispaire, and lament, when no cause requireth it, but rather a behauiour beseeminge a heart vppon
iust

iust cause, and sound reason most comfortable, and chearfull. This doth melancholie work, not otherwise then the former humours, giuing occasion, and false matter of these passions, and not by any disposition as of instrument thereunto. Of all the other humours melancholie is fullest of varietie of passion, both according to the diuersitie of place where it setleth, as brayne, splene, mesaraicke vaines, hart, womb, and stomach; as also through the diuerse kindes, as naturall, vnnaturall: naturall, either of the splene, or of the vaines, faultie only by excesse of quantitie, or thicknesse of substance: vnnaturall by corruption, and that either of bloud adust, choler, or melancholie naturall, by excessiue distemper of heate, turned in comparison of the naturall, into a sharpe lye by force of adustion. These diuerse sorts hauing diuerse matter, cause mo straunge symptomes of fancie and affection to melancholike persons, then their humour to such as are sanguine, cholericke, or flegmaticke: which fleume of all the rest serueth least to stir vp any affection: but breeding rather a kind of stupiditie, and an impassionate hart, then easily moued to embrace or refuse, to sorowe or ioye, anger or contentednesse: except it be a salte fleume, thē approcheth it to the natur of choler, & in like sort therof riseth anger & frowardnes.

CHAP. XVII.
How melancholy procureth feare, sadnes, dispaire, and such other passions.

NOw let vs consider what passions they are that melancholy driueth vs vnto, and the reason how it doth so diuersly distract those that are oppressed therewith. The perturbations of melancholy are for the most parte, sadde and fearefull, and such as rise of them: as distrust, doubt, diffidence, or dispaire, sometimes furious, and sometimes merry in apparaunce, through a kinde of Sardoniā, and false laughter, as the humour, is disposed that procureth these diuersities. Those which are sad and pensiue, rise of that melancholick humour, which is the grossest part of the blood, whether it be iuice or excrement, not passing the naturall temper in heat whereof it partaketh, and is called cold in comparison onely. This for the most part is setled in the spleane, and with his vapours anoyeth the harte and passing vp to the brayne, counterfetteth terible obiectes to the fantasie, and polluting both the substance, and spirits of the brayne, causeth it without externall occasiō, to forge monstrous fictions, and terrible to the conceite, which the iudgement taking as they are presented by the disordered instrument, deliuer ouer to the hart, which hath no iudgement of discretion in it self, but giuing credite to the mistaken report of the braine, breaketh out into that inordinate passion, against reason. This commeth to passe, because the instrument of discretion is deprauved by these melancholick spirites, and a darknes & cloudes of melancholievapours rising from that pudle of the splene obscure the clearenes, which our spirites are endued with, and is requisite to the due discretion of outward obiectes. This at the first is not so extreame, neither doth it shew

OF MELANCHOLIE. 103

so apparauntly, as in processe of time, when the substance of the brayne hath plentifully drunke of that spleneticke fogge, whereby his nature is become of the same quality, and the pure and bright spirites so defiled, and eclipsed, that their indifferency alike to all sensible thinges, is now drawen to a partiality, and inclination, as by melancholy they are inforced. For where that naturall and internall light is darkened, their fansies arise vayne, false, and voide of ground: euen as in the externall sensible darkenes, a false illusion will appeare vnto our imagination, which the light being brought in is discerned to be an abuse of fancie: now the internall darknes affecting more nigh by our nature, then the outward, is cause of greater feares, and more molesteth vs with terror, then that which taketh from vs the sight of sensible thinges: especially arising not of absence of light only, but by a presence of a substantiall obscurity, which is possessed with an actuall power of operation: this taking hold of the brayne by processe of time giueth it an habite of depraued conceite, whereby it fancieth not according to truth: but as the nature of that humour leadeth it, altogether gastely and fearefull. This causeth not only phantasticall apparitions wrought by apprehēsion only of common sense, but fantasie, an other parte of internall sense compoundeth, and forgeth disguised shapes, which giue great terror vnto the heart, and cause it with the liuely spirit to hide it selfe as well as it can, by contraction in all partes, from those counterfet goblins, which

G iiij

the brayne dispossessed of right discerning, sayneth vnto the heart. Neither only is common sense, and fantasie thus ouertaken with delusion, but memory also receiueth a wound therewith: which disableth it both to keepe in memory, and to record those thinges, whereof it tooke some custody before this passion, and after, therewith are defaced. For as the common sense and fantasie, which doe offer vnto the memory to lay vp, deliuer but fables in stead of true report, and those tragicall that dismay all the sensible frame of our bodies, so eyther is the memory wholly distract by importunity of those doubtes and feares, that it neglecteth the custody of other store: or else it recordeth and apprehendeth only such as by this importunity is thrust therupon nothing but darkenes, perill, doubt, frightes, and whatsoeuer the harte of man most doth abhor. And these the senses do so melancholikely deliuer to the mindes consideration (which iudging of such thinges as they offered, not hauing farther to do in the deeper examination) that it applyeth those certayne ingenerate pointes of reason and wisedome to a deceitfull case, though it be alwayes in the generall, and if particularities be deliuered vp a right, in them also most certaine and assured. For those thinges which are sensible, and are as it were the counterfettes of outward creatures, the reporte of them is committed by Gods ordinaunce to the instruments of the brayne furnished with his spirite, which if it be, as the thinges are in nature, so doth the minde iudge and determine, no farther submitting

ting it selfe to examine the credite of these senses which (the instrumentes being saultles, and
certaine other considerations required necessary, agreeable vnto their integrity,) neuer faile in
their busines, but are the very first groundes of
all this corporall action of life and wisedome,
that the minde for the most parte here outwardly practileth. If they be contrary, so also doth the
minde iudge, and pursueth or shuneth, for these
sensible matters reposing trust in the corporall
ministers, whose misereport, no more ought to
discredite the minde, or draw it into an accessa-
ry crime of error, then the iudiciall sentence is
to be blamed, which pronounceth vpon the oth
and credite of a iurie impanelled of such as are
reported men of honesty, credite, and discretion
though their verdict be not peraduenture according as the cause committed to them doth
require. The memory being thus fraight with
perills past: and embracing only through the
braynes disorder that which is of discomforte,
causeth the fantasie out of such recordes, to
forge new matters of sadnes and feare, whereof
no occasion was at any time before, nor like to
be giuen hereafter: to these fansies the hart answering with like melancholicke affection, turneth all hope into feare, assurance into distrust
and dispaire, ioye into discomforte: and as the
melancholie nature, or bodie any waie corrupt,
defileth the pure and holesome nourishment, &
conuerteth it into the same kinde of impuritie:
and as the fire of all kinde of matter giueth increase of heate, whether it be wood, stone, metal,

or liquor: so the body thus possessed with the vnchearefull, and discomfortable darknes of melácholie, obscureth the Sonne and Moone, and all the comfortable planetts of our natures, in such sort, that if they appeare, they appeare all darke, and more then halfe eclipsed of this mist of blackenes, rising from that hidious lake: and in all thinges comfortable, either curiously pryeth out, and snatcheth at whatsoeuer of mislike may be drawen to the nourishment of it selfe: or else neglecteth altogether that which is of other qualitie, then foode, and pasture of those monsters, which nature neuer bred, nor perfect since conceiued, nor memorie vncorrupt would euer allow entertainement, but are hatched out of this muddie humour, by an vnnaturall temper & bastard spirite, to the disorder of the whole regiment of humane nature, both in iudgement and affection. Thus the hart a while being acquainted, with nothing else, but domesticall terror, feareth euery thing, and the brayne simpathetically partaking with the hartes feare, maketh doubt, distrusteth, & suspecteth without cause, alwayes standing in awe of grieuaunce: wherwith in time it becommeth so tender, that the least touch, as it were ones naile in an vlcer, giueth discouragement thereto, rubbing it vpon the gale exulcerate with sorow and feare: neither only doubleth it sorrow vpon smal occasion, but taketh it where none is offered: euen as the Cholerick man feedeth his passió with ridiculous causes of displeasure. For first (the generall being in al natures actions before the particular) the heart by the braine

Of Melancholie. 107

braine solicited to passiō, & vsed to grief & feare, taketh the accustomed way of flight and auoydance, abhorring & fearing those thinges, which of themselues are most amiable and gratefull: at the first not being aduised, whereto to apply the passion: euen as one condemned to death with vndoubted expectation of execution, fearing euerie knock at the prison doore, hath horrour, though the messenger of pardon with knock require to be admitted & let in, and euery messenger, where daunger is feared, though he come with cherefull countenance, giueth cause of distrust when there may be assurance: euen so, the heart ouercome with inward heauines, and skared with inward feares, faireth as though whatsoeuer cause of affection and perturbation were minister of present griefe, or messenger of future daunger, by mistaking only, and withdraweth it selfe, and shroudeth it as secrete and closse, as nature will suffer, from that, which if custome had not bent it another way, vppon aduisement (now banished through swiftnes and vhemēcy of passion) it would haue with ioyful cheare embraced. For euē as we se in outward sense: the ey, or the eare long and vehemently affected with colour, or sound, or the nose with strong sent: retaine the verie colour, sound, and sent in the instrumentes, though the thing be remoued that yeelded such qualities; so the internall senses molested continually with this fearefull obiect of internall darknes, esteemeth euery thing of that nature: the true qualitie thereof being obscure, by that which hath taken possession of the before. The brayne thus affected, and the heart anſwering his paſſion thereafter driueth vs into thoſe extremities of heauy moôde, which aſſaile and diſpoſſeſſe of right vſe of reaſon thoſe who are melancholickly diſpoſed: much more if the heart be as melancholickly bent, as the brayne: then diuerſe times doth it preuent the fancie with feare, and as a man tranſported with paſſiõ is vtterly bereft of aduiſemẽt, cauſeth the ſenſes both outward & inward prepoſterouſly to conceiue, as the heart vainely feareth. This melancholy as the parts are diuerſe, & actions vary, ſo doth it as it is ſeated, or paſſeth this or that way, breed diuerſity of paſſion: as in the heart a trembling, in the ſtomach a greedy appetite: in the brayne falſe illuſions, and in the other partes as they are diſpoſed: ſo deprauing their actions, it cauſeth much variety of effects, which are not in the nature of the humor, but as it diſturbeth the actiue inſtrumentes, no more then darknes cauſeth ſome to ſtũble, other ſome to go out of their way, & wander, & other ſome to bringe to paſſe ſuch purpoſes, as light would bewray & hinder, al as they be diſpoſed & occupied w̃ take thẽ to their buſines in the dark, & not through any ſuch effectuall operatiõ of darkenes, which is naught elſe but meere abſence of light. Neither doth ſo many ſtraunge ſortes of accidentes follow melãcholie through diuerſity of parts only: but as the cuſtome of life hath bene before, & the fancie, & heart ſome way vehemently occupied: there through this humour all the faculties afore named, are carried the ſame way, as it were with the

the streame of a tide, driuen with a boysterous wind; which causeth that melancholicke men, are not all of one nature passionate this way: the one taking his dolorous passion from his loue, an other from his wealth: the other frō his pleasures, whereof his melancholie beareth him in hand the present losse, or imminent daunger of that wherein affection in former times had surest footing: & on the other part, which before a man most abhorred, that nowe the humor vrgeth with most vehemencie. Againe as it is mixed with other humours, either keeping mediocrity, or abounding; so likewise breaketh it forth into such diuersities, & manie times into plaine contrarieties of conceit and perturbation. Thus you vnderstand, howe feares and sorowes rise, without cause from naturall melancholie, whether it be iuyce, or excrement, not through chiefe action, as from worke of facultie, but by abuse of instrument through occasion. If the spleneticke excrement surcharge the bodie, not being purged by helpe of the splene: then are these perturbations farre more outragious, and harde to be mitigated by counsell or perswasion: and more do they enforce vs, the partes being altered with corporall humour, then with spirituall vapour: and so are the passions longer in continuance, and more extreeme in vehemencie. For as the flame carrieth not such force of burning as the cole, neither contayneth the heate so longe; euen so the partes affected with the humour, which carrieth both grossenesse of substance, with continuall supplie of that dimme vapour, settleth a more fixed passion of feare and heauinesse, then that which riseth from the vapour onely, partly of the owne accorde more easily vanishing and partly with greater facillitie wasted by natures strife and resistance. Nowe it followeth to declare, howe the other vnnaturall melancholy annoyeth with passions, & abuseth vs with coūterfet cause of perturbation, whereof there is no ground in truth, but onely a vaine and fantasticall conceit.

Chap. XVIII.
Of the vnnaturall melancholie rising by adustion, how it affecteth vs with diuers passions.

Besides the former kindes, there are sortes of vnnaturall melancholie: which I call so rather then the other, bicause the other offendeth onely in qualitie, or quantitie: these are of another nature farre disagreeing from the other, & by an vnproper speech called melancholy. They rise of the naturall humors, or their excrements by excessiue distēper of heate, burned as it were into ashes in comparison of humour, by which the humour of like nature being mixed, turneth it into a sharp lye: sanguine, cholericke, or melancholicke, according to the humour thus burned, which we call by name of melancholie. This sort raiseth the greatest tempest of perturbatiōs and most of all destroyeth the braine with all his faculties, and disposition of action, and maketh both it, & the hart cheere more vncomfortably:

and

Of Melancholie.

and if it rise of the naturall melancholy, beyond all likelihood of truth, frame monst.ous terrors of feare and heauinesse without cause. If it rise of choler, then rage playeth her part, and furie ioyned with madnesse, putteth all out of frame. If bloud minister matter to this fire, euery serious thing for a time, is turned into a iest, & tragedies into comedies, and lamentation into gigges and daunces: thus the passion whereof the humour min streth occasion by this vnkindly heate aduaunceth it selfe into greater extremities. For becomming more subtile by heate, both in substance, & spirit, it passeth more deeply into all the parts of the instrument it selfe, and is a conueyance also to the humour of the same kind: making away for naturall melancholie, wherewith it is mixed, into the verie inward secrets of those instruments, wherof passions are affected, euen hart and braine. Thus affected, you haue men, when desperate furie is ioyned with feare: which so terrifieth, that to auoid the terrour, they attempt sometimes to depriue thē selues of life: so irksome it is vnto them through these tragicall conceits, although waighing and considering death by it self without comparison, and force of the passion, none more feare it thē they. These most seeke to auoyde the society of men, and betake them to wildernesses, and deserts, finding matter of feare in euery thing they behold, and best at ease, when alone they may digest these fancies without new prouocations, which they apprehende in humane societie. If choller haue yeelded matter to this sharpe kind of melancholie, then rage, reuenge, and furie, possesse both hart and head, and the whole bodie is caried with that storme, contrarie to persuasion of reason: which hath no farther power ouer these affections, then by way of counsell to giue other direction (whereof the hart it selfe is destitute) and taking these discomfortes of the credit of the senses, according thereto it applieth it selfe, working, and disposing the ingenerate wisedome it is indued with, vnto these particulars, which the corporall instruments corruptly offer vnto it: which ministreth doubt and question to some not well aduised in this point, whether reason it selfe be not impaired by these corporall alterations, and the immortall & impatible mind hereby suffreth not violence; which is farre otherwise, if we duly way the matter. For the mad man, of what kinde soeuer he be of, as truly concludeth of that which fantasie ministreth of conceit, as the wisest: onely therein lieth the abuse and defect, that the organicall parts which are ordained embassadours, & notaries vnto the mind in these cases, falsifie the report, and deliuer corrupt recordes. This is to be helped, as it shall be declared more at large hereafter, by counsell only sincerely ministred, which is free from the corruptions of those officers, and deliuereth truth vnto the mind, wherby it putteth in practise contrary to these importunate and furious sollicitors. This furie is bred, because choler thus adust, getteth a greater egernesse of qualitie, and molesting the inward parts, and toyling the spirits, ingendreth a

greater

Of Melancholie.

greater inwarde disquiet and discontentment, then cruder choler doth procure. The third sort is of merie melãcholie, which riseth of the bloud ouer heated in such sort as I haue declared. Of all the rest of humours, bloud is most temperat and mild of disposition, and comforteth the bodie, as hath bene mentioned, whose substaunce receauing that burning heat, whereof riseth the third kind of this vnnaturall melancholie, procureth it to be of a nature quicke and fresh, and indueth it with a spirite of a nature somewhat more itching, and as it were, of a tickling qualitie then bloud it selfe. For of it selfe being (if it be pure and perfect) nutsweete, or milkesweete, by this heate becommeth first suger or hony sweet, which hath more force of affecting, and obtayneth a more subtile and quicke spirit: afterward by operation of heate, this sweetnesse is conuerted into a mild saltnesse, voyd of fretting, which tickling and itching in these melancholicke bodies, cause them rather to be giuen to a ridiculous and absurd meriment, then a sound ioye of hart, and comfortable gladnesse: which forceth them into laughter somtimes, that without ceasing, to the tyring and wearying of their bodies, no perswasion of reason is able to call them to more sobrietie. We may see in boyling of milke, what sweetnesse is procured vnto it thereby: & howe hony much boyled, becometh salt & bitter: such is the force of heat in bloud, that it turneth that milke sweet tast, into hony sweet: and that into a gentle & itching brackishnes, whereby the melancholicke bodies, being as it were tickled, render from their foolish fantasie, and false liking of the hart, many absurd and ridiculous gestures and speeches, and (as farre'altered this way, as the melancholick on the other side) snatch at smal occasions, or none at all ofttimes, of answering this fond humor in outward lightnesse of gesture & countenance. Thus you heare in what sort the humoures seeme to affect the mind, euerie one singled and keeping apart from his other fellowe humours: which, as they be tempered with the other naturall, or compounded together with one or twaine of the like vnnaturall sortes of melancholie, make many distinctions, and differences of melancholie passions: as some more sadde, the other some more merie, some quieter, & other some more prone to rage and furie: and as the humors haue their courses, as for the yeare, bloud in the spring, choller in sommer, melancholie in autumne, & fleume in winter: for the houre according to Soranus Ephesius opinion, bloud from three of the clocke in the morning, till nine of the same day, choler from nine of the morning, till three at afternoone, melancholie frō 3. at after noone till nine at night, and fleume from nine at night til the third of the morning. I say if a man obserue all these varieties, by mixture, and season, with inclination of the partes, custome of life, and imbecillitie of some part, and proportionallie match the multitude of passions with these occasions, he might haue the grounde of all these troublesome perturbations made playne vnto him: why some are contrarie affected to other

some

some in their melancholicke fits, and are not all times alike, but sometimes sad, and sometimes excessiue in mirth, now more outragious, then at another time, as season of the yeare, and time of the day approch, wherein these humors haue more speciall and perticuler operation. But it were too long to descend into such particularities: it shall suffice only, to haue declared howe these humors become occasions of passions vnto vs, and to haue noted such a generalitie of rule, as any one may with ease thereby discipher the particulars. By that which hitherto hath bin shewed, it appeareth these humours only affect the organ and corporall part, & nothing come nigh the mind and soule: which in the meane time of these stormes and tempests of passion, these delusions, feares, false terrours, and poeticall fictions of the braine, sitteth quiet and still, nothing altered in facultie, or any part of that diuine and impatible disposition, which it obtaineth by the excellencie of creation: no more then the Sunne is moued in the heauens, or receaueth in it selfe an obscuritie, when stormes arise, thunder, lightning, and cloudes of darkenesse, and boysterous whirlewindes, seeme here belowe to mixe heauen and earth together, and to make confusion in the course and frame of nature. And thus haue you the obiections aleaged against that freedome of the soule from the inconueniences, aunswered I trust to your contentment. Diuerse accidents followe these humours, which are to be shewed, both of fansie, sense, and affection, and also gestures & actions of weeping, sighing, sobbing, laughing, & such like, with the reasons of ech one, and howe they be wrought by these passions: which I deferre in this place to discusse, being called on to prosecute the aunswer to the rest of the doubts propounded before: which done (that nothing, so farre as my vnderstanding & memorie will help to the matter, may be leaft obscure vnto you in this case of melancholie) I will hereafter prosecute those also, as I shall haue done the causes from whence they proceede.

Chap. XIX.

Howe sickenesse and yeares seeme to alter the minde: and the cause: and how the soule hath practise of senses, being separated from the bodie.

Although persons so disposed with melancholie (as hath bene declared) enioy not perfect estate of health, yet because they complaine not, neither are accompted sicke, neither lye for the matter, but seeme (their fancies and vaine feares excepted) to be otherwise healthfull, I so take them in this place though their bodie be in that sort, as I haue mentioned to be charged with defect, as vnsound and imperfect. The last of the obiections is taken frō the condition of sicke persons, who as in apparance it seemeth both receaue in their mindes alteration of defect, and increase of faculties through the corporall imbecillitie: as though at certaine times the bodies health were transported to the esta-

OF MELANCHOLIE.

establishment of the mind, or the bodie at other times, & after another sort weake, did communicate that also vnto the soule, as disburthening it selfe thereon. To which obiection, the general aunswer of organicall disposition of parts is here more particularly to be applied: & as in the former doubtes, so in this I iudge all such actions, as the mind seemeth to performe in that state of bodie, better or worse, to be organicall, pertinent to sensible things: & which as it practiseth not but in this life, neither hath such vse of being disioyned from this masse of earth whereto it is with spirite coupled, so in her faculties she is not to be esteemed subiect to these alteratiōs. But you demaund a farther declaration of this point, whether the minde hath vse of sense or not, after it dislodgeth from this earthly tabernacle. To satisfie you herein, if probabilitie of reason will serue, I do not take it otherwise, then that it is all an eye, all an eare, all nose, tast and sinewe, without distinction, as these seuerall instruments which nowe it employeth make shew of: For then were it not simple in substance, but must needs haue compounded substance, to answer these particular senses. If you require experience and example of this, because it cannot be had in soules departed (but reason onely vpholdeth the rule in respect of them) let vs take that which dreames in sleep do minister for declaration of this point, which sleepe is a kind of separation of the soule from the body for a time, at the least a rest from outward sensible actions, whereby it more freely applyeth it selfe to those

H iij

diuine contemplations, which is onely learned from the instinct of creatiō, & neuer apprehended by any other instruction. In sleep I say, our dreames in some sort make euident vnto vs, how the soule without instrument, lacketh not the practise of senses: in which dreames we see with our soules, heare, talke, conferre, and practise what action soeuer, as euidently with affection of ioye or sorowe, as if the very object of these senses were represented vnto vs brode awake at noone day. If you will say it is nothing else, but the images of outward thinges, which hang in the common sense presented to the fantasie, or offered of the memorie, which inward senses are alwayes watchfull when the outward take rest: how then commeth it to passe, that we can not in like sort fancie being awake? If we shold striue to do it, euery one should find it impossible, as I take it: because the soule is in a sorte by that great law of necessitie (being chained with that golden chaine) in all parts linked to this bodie, which being awake, letteth those sincere actions whereabout it is busied in sleepe: wherein euery dreame seemeth to be a kind of extasie, or traunce, & separation of the soule from this bodily societie, in which it hath bene in olde time instructed of God by reuelation, and misteries of secrets reuealed vnto it, as then more fit to apprehend such diuine oracles, then altogether enioying awake the corporall societie of these earthly members. But you will say such dreames are oft times but fancies. True: and many times they be no fancies; whereof infinite examples

may

may be brought, both sacred & prophane. Now when they be not, sufficient profe ariseth to that I nowe dispute, that soules haue sense of thinges without organicall senses: and when they be but fancies, yet that which ministreth the obiect, from some distemper of diet, or condition of the bodie, good or bad, is sented with the mind only, the outward senses being all in deepe sleepe, and the inwarde hauing no power at all to see, heare, smell, tast or feele, but only of discerning that which the outward sense deliuereth: for third, there is none to whome these actions are to be ascribed. Neither are these sensible actions of the minde to be accempted false: because it seeth in dreames things past as present: for so it doth also future things sometimes: which rather may argue, that both past, and to come are both present vnto the mind, of such things as fall into the capacitie of her consideration. If anie man thinke it much to aduaunce the mind so high, let him remember from whom it proceeded, & the maner howe it was created, and the most excellent estate thereof before the fall, and no doubt it will sufficiently aunswer that difficultie, and confirme that which I haue said. And thus much for that interruption of my aunswer to the obiection from sicknesse: whether the soule hath outward sense and not organicall, or no. Now to prosecute the aunswere: I say all those which seeme to be faculties altered in sicknesses, be only organicall dispositions which the soule vseth as she findeth them. As for the outward senses, the humidities, and superfluities of the eares in

H iiij

some sickneffe being dried vp, maketh hearing more quicke then in health: so the poores of smelling may be more open: and the eye by the same reason receaue quicker sight: and the sense of feeling more exact: or by reason the spirites are more subtile, which thereby with greater ease flowe into all partes of the inftrument nowe emptied of superfluity. Againe in phrenticke persons, we see through drinesse of the braine and sinewes, what strength they become of, that sower men in health are scarse able to hold them, though otherwise weake and feeble Nowe the outward passages of senses thus cleared, and the spirits more rare and subtile, deliuer more exactly to the inwarde the Ideas of such things as require to be admitted: which inward senses by like disposition of the braine, more exactly discerne the outward qualitie of thinges, & deliuer more sincere reporte vnto the minde, which finding all so cleare giueth sentence, pronounceth, and debateth more perfectly, in respect of that distinction and clearnesse it findeth in those personall representations of thinges; which may seeme vnto such as consider not duely whereof it riseth, to be an increase of gift in the minde by sickenesse, and not greater clearenesse of the obiect. This disposition of instrument causeth some children to be more pregnant then other some, and in sickenesse manie one to be of better aduisement then in health: and if you list inferre it vppon the former g oundes; I will not denie this to be the cause whie some be idiottes and fooles, and

other

Of Melancholie.

other some of quicke spirit, and prompt witted. Nowe as this clearing of the poores, and subtiliation of spirits, is cause of these more readie and distinct actions in sicknesse then in health, and in youth aboue the tendernesse of yeares: so in health the poores replenished with their humours, and the spirites recouering their ordinarie grossenesse, or mediocritie, the actions become of the same condition they were before: not by anie alteration of facultie, but through instrument diuersly disposed. In like manner the aged, farre stroken in yeares, faile in the execution of externall actions: though their mindes should rather be wiser through experience, (if anie thing be learned by the practise of this life) by excrementitious humiditie, and rewmaticke superfluities, which drowne the instrument; and an internal drinesse, wherby all wayes to that small rénant of spirit is stopped, through contraction and shrinking of poores, the verie cundites of the spirit into all the corporal members: neither only do they faile in outward sense and motion, but by the internall also suffer like imbecillitie, whereuppon their minde framinge conclusions vpon false groundes, seeme to faile in that action also, not hauing better matter to work on. If you say vnto me: why is not this helped by that inorganicall sense of the minde, and so these inconueniences auoyded? you must cõsider the minde neuer exerciseth that, but being withdrawen from the corporall socie y, & these mechanicall actions, which in a maner in sleepe & extasie it is: then it maketh choice of particulars, as it listeth it selfe: what, who, where, and when: neither is it tied to these outward ministers, or those Ideas which they take viewe of. Moreouer we must remember that during this life (sauing vpon certaine occasions extraordinary,) God hath ordained these actions corporal: neither is it necessary that wants of outward senses should be so supplied, which (before sinne tooke such hold of soule and body) were not subiect to these imbecillities, but perfectly and sincerely deliuered the condition of sensible things to the mindes consideration, which reposing trust in them, according to the integrity wherin they first stoode, dischargeth her office of vnderstãding, iudging, and willing, as this way only it findeth cause. And thus much touching the aunswere to the former obiections: notwithstanding whose probabilities to the contrary, you may perceiue how the body only receiueth these alterations before mentioned, euen as instruments of a corporall substance, and raised from the earth, subiect to earthly and elementary chaunges, without touch of soule, or disturbing of that immortal nature, which proceeded from the breath of God, and is of a more noble race: neither are you so to vnderstand me, as though I accompted the soule in this present state equall with the first creation: that were erronious and against the history of mãs fall, and of that curse, which ensued through disobedience, and contrary to that experience, which euery one findeth of imbecillity in the most excellent actions of the minde, and such as require no organ: but

my

my discourse tendeth in this point to exempt it from corporal contagion only, which it can not in any sort receiue, more then the heauens pollution from the earth, being a nature farre more different in comparison then the heauens, from this inferiour world, which is alotted to our vse of habitation. Hauing hitherto declared how perturbations rise of humors, although it be not greatly pertinent to the matter in hand, of coūsell, in this passion: yet because my meaning is not only to satisfie your request in that, but also to giue you argumēt of philosophicall discourse, to occupie your selfe in this heauy time, wherein both melancholie doth all it may to discourage you, and Sathan the old enimy taketh aduantage to serue his turne vpō your present imbecillity, I will add the reason of such accidentes as fall vnto these passions, in such probability, as my habilitie will affoord, both for mine owne exercise, aud your contentment, whom in times past I haue knowen to be delighted with studie of philosophie.

Chap. XX.

The accidenses which befall melancholicke persons.

AS all other state of bodie, so the melancholick sheweth it self, either in the qualities of the body, or in the deeds. Of the qualities which are first taken frō the elemēts, the melācholick without adustion, is cold and drie: of such as are second, rising from the first, of colour blacke and swart, of substance inclyning to hardnes, leane, and spare of flesh: which causeth hollownes of eye, and vnchearefulnes of countenance, all these more or lesse, some or all: either as the melancholy is ingenerate, or gotten by error of diet, hath continued longer, or short time. Of deedes, and such as are actions of the brayne, either of sense and motions, dull, both in outward senses, and conceite. Of memory reasonable good, if fancies deface it not: firme in opinion, and hardly remoued wher it is resolued: doubtfull before, and long in deliberation: suspicious, painefull in studie, and circumspect, giuen to fearefull and terrible dreames: in affection sad, & full of feare hardly moued to anger, but keeping it long, and not easie to be reconciled: enuious, and ielous, apt to take occasions in the worse part, and out of measure passionate, whereto it is moued. Frō these two dispositions of brayne and heart arise solitarines, morning, weeping, & (if it be of sanguine adust) melancholic laughter, sighing, sobbing, lamentation, countenance demisse, and hanging downe, blushing and bashfull, of pace slow, silent, negligent, refusing the light and frequency of men, delighted more in solitarines & obscurity. These are actiōs which lie in our powers to doe, and are called animall. Of naturall actions, their appetite is of greater then their concoction, digestion slow, and excretion not so ready, pulse rare, and slow. And thus faireth it with melancholy persons in those deedes which are actions. Other deedes are certayne workes,

and

Of Melancholie.

and effectes of their naturall actions: such are nutritiue iuice, or excrement. Their nutritiue iuice as blood, and the secondary humours that rise there from, are thick and grosse, their blood blacke, and nothing fresh. Their melancholicke excrement very much, if the splene do his part: if it faile, either by imbecillity of attraction, or any hinderance of obstruction, then is it more plentifull in the vaynes, and greately altereth the complexion: if it discharge not .t felfe of the superfluitie of that it hath drawen frō the blood, then swelleth it, and groweth it into obstructions, causeth shortnes of breathing, especially after meate, and an vnnaturall boyling of heate, with wyndines vnder the left side, and plenty of humidity in the stomach, which aboundeth in spitting by hindering the first concoction in the stomach and noysome vapours, causing palpitation of the heart. The excrement of stoole is hard, blacke, and seeldome: vrine pale, and verie low coloured, nor much in quantitie. These are the chiefe accidentes which fall vnto melácholicke persons: of them I will deliuer vnto you the particular causes, so farre as belongeth vnto the charge of this melancholicke discourse.

Chap. XXI.
How melancholy altereth the quallities of the body.

THE bodies of melancholike persons, if they be naturally giuen to that humor, or otherwyse it hath preuailed in time vpon them, are

colder, and dryer then others, or if they be such by error of diet, thē in times past they théselues haue bene: partly through contagion of that humor, which with his cold altereth the complexion, and partly by the nourishment taken from the masse of blood: becaufe all the partes are maintayned, and releeued with cold and dry aliment, the rest of the blood being cooled by that grosse, and earthy parte. Sometimes it faireth with them otherwise, to be intemperately hote through obstruction, which may gather heat in the splene, and so accidentally breed an hoate distemper. Againe if the melancholie be of the adust kinde, which pertaketh of heate, and becommeth eger and fell, then are they also distēpered in heate, or at the least not molested with cold, and howsoeuer it faire with them in hoate or cold, alwayes they keepe drie in substance of their bodies, both the naturall, and the adust amelancholy agreeing therewith. An humidity they haue of Rewme, and spitting from the stomach, whose concoction is hindred, and natural heate cooled sometimes by the splenes disorder, which lieth nigh thereunto, and may with more plenty then need requireth of that soure iuice, which serueth to stirre vp appetite, dull that heat of the stomach wherewith the concoction is made perfect, and excrementes become few: but this is a moistnes excrementitious, and accidentall in that parte, and peraduenture like in the brayne, by consent of the stomach: the substance of the rest keeping drie through the nature of the nourishment, which in time maketh

OF MELANCHOLIE.

keth the complexion of like qualitie. They are not so well flesht, nor in such good plight, as either they haue ben, or as some other complexion: by reason all the natural actions, that should serue that vse, are become weaker, & as it were smothered with this soote of melancholie: neither is the melancholie blood cold and drie, a fitte matter to raise vp fatt, or plenty of flesh: for to both these are requisite a moderatiō of complexiō in the first qualities, and a matter of moderate temper, which may entertaine both flesh and fat. Thirdly the poores of the body being not so free, for distribution of blood, by reason of their grosse nourishment, and nature of the humor with which his coldnes and sowernes, (for such is the taste of melancholie) closeth vp the poores, or straightneth the passages, & of it selfe also slow of mouing, the bodie can not be filled with that corpulency which falleth to other cōplexions. To the nourishment and good plight of the body, these three are necessarie: cōplexion temperat, matter moderat, and passage free: which all falling contrary in melancholick persons, hindereth them of that good liking, & fullnes of body, which otherwise they might enioy. For if the complexiō be too hote then wasteth it, and therein riseth the cholerick skreetnes: if it be too cold, then raiseth it not sufficiency of nourishment of meates, drinckes, & whatsoeuer we vse for sustentatiō of life: but leaueth it crude and maketh mo superfluities. If it be drie, then drinketh it vp vnto the solide partes, that which should baste and line the body with, hauing not to spare. If moist, then in stead of firme substāce, the body is ouercharged with a counterfette kinde of fatte, and hydropical rogge, which beareth shewe of good habite. If the matter be hoat or drie, it soone vanitheth, or hath not that store of nourishing iuice, to yeeld matter of flesh and fatte, besides the firme nourishment. If moyst, then swelleth it the body: and as water enlargeth a sponge, so doth moist nourishment soake into the bodie, and beareth it out, as fast substance doth naturally fill, raised from temperate nourishmēt. If cold, then both hath it small portion of naturall iuice, and slow to be passed from parte to parte, it is not easily receiued into euery member, where of corpulencie doth rise. The passages being either narrow of themselues, or hindered by stopping, distribution is likewise letted, very requisite to the maintenance of good liking, and moderate habite of the body: which being ouerlarge giue entertainement and place to grossenes, whether it be sound, or in apparance. Now these three falling out, cold, drie, thick and hard of passage, in melancholick persons, procure that leane, and spare bodie of the melancholicke: except it be by former custome of diet, or naturally otherwise, which the force of melancholy hath not yet so farre altered. Of this coldnes and drynes, riseth hardnes whereof the flesh of melancholy persons is: except the melancholy rise of some disorder of diet, or passions, and hath not yet entred so farre vpon the complexion. Of colour they be black, according to the humour whereof they are nourished, and

the

the skinne alwayes receauing the blacke vapors, which insensibly do passe from the inward parts, taketh die and staine thereof: sauing that in the beginning it may come to passe otherwise, the body white, and bloud blacke; nature for a time seruing her selfe of that which is purest, and leauing the grossest in the vaines, till for want of better, in the end it be faine to take of the melancholicke, which before it disdained: then altereth it the colour, and fairenesse is turned into morphe, maketh euident the humour which gaue the die, & hath obscured the former beautie. And thus are the qualities of melancholie bodies altered by this grosse, earthie and darke humour.

Chap. XXII.
How melancholie altereth those actions which rise out of the braine.

Touching actions which rise from the brain, melancholie causeth dulnesse of conceit, both by reason the substance of the braine in such personnes is more grosse, and their spirite not so prompt and subtile as is requisit for readie vnderstandinge. Againe almost all the senses standing in a kinde of passiue nature, a substance cold and drie, and by consequent hard, is not so meete thereto; which as it serueth well to retaine that which is once ingrauen, so like adamant it keepeth, in comparison of other tempers, that which once it hath receaued: whereby as they are vnfit to commit readily to memorie, so retaine they that is committed in surer custodie. Sometime it falleth out, that melancholie men are found verie wittie, and quickly discerne: either because the humour of melancholie with some heate is so made subtile, that as from the driest woode riseth the clearest flame, and from the lyes of wine is distilled a strong & burning aqua vitæ, in like sort their spirits, both from the drinesse of the matter, and straining of the grosse substance from which they passe, receauing a purenesse, are instrumentes of such sharpnesse: which is the drie light that Heraclitus approued. To this, other reasons may be added: as exercise of their wittes, wherein they be indefatigable: which maketh them seeme to haue that of a naturall readinesse, which custome of exercise, and vse hath found in them. Moreouer, while their passions be not yet vehemēt, whereby they might be ouercaried, melancholy breedeth a ielousie of doubt in that they take in deliberation, and causeth them to be the more exact & curious in pōdering the very moments of things: to these reasons may be added, the vehemencie of theyr affection once raysed: which carieth them, with all their faculties therto belonging, into the deapth of that they take pleasure to intermeddle in. For though the melancholie man be not so easily affected with any other passion, as with those of feare, sadnesse,& ielosie, yet being once throughly heat with a cōtrarie passion, retaineth the feruency thereof farre longer time then anie other complexion: and more feruently boyleth therewith, by reason his heart and spirite hath more solliditie of

substance

Of Melancholie.

substance to entertayne deepely the passion, which in a more rare and thinne sooner vanisheth away. Thus greedinesse of desire in those thinges which they affect, maketh them diligent and painefull, warie and circumspect, and so in actions of braine and sense not inferiour to the best tempers; as also it maketh them stiffe in opinion. Their resolution riseth of long deliberation, because of doubt and distrust: which as it is not easily bred, so it is also harde to remoue. Such persons are doubtfull, suspitious, and thereby long in deliberation, because those domesticall feares, or that internall obscuritie, causeth an opinion of daunger in outwarde affaires, where there is no cause of doubt: their dreames are fearefull: partly by reason of their fancie waking, is most occupied about feares, and terrours, which retayneth the impression in sleepe, and partly through blacke and darke fumes of melancholie, rising vp to the braine, whereof the fantasie forgeth obiectes, and disturbeth the sleep of melancholy persons. These persons are also subiect to that kinde of suffocation in the night, which is called the mare, wherein, with some horrible vision in dreame they are halfe strangled, and intercepted of speech, through they striue to call. This happeneth through grosse melancholicke vapours in them which cause horrible and fearefull apparitions, by reason of the nature of that humour, and the fancie prone through custome to conteaue on the worse parte, and stoppeth theyr winde, by occupying the passages of such spirits

I ij

as rise from the braine, and flowe into the nerues which serue certaine muscles of respiration: it happeneth chiefly when they lye on their backe, and somewhat too low with their heade; because both the midriffe (a chiefe muscle of respiration) is more pressed with the bowelles, which lye vnder it, the stomach is not so firmely closed, whereby vapours more easily haue vent, and the whole bulke of the chest in that position of the bodie, lying more heauily vppon them, requireth greater force of mouing facultie, whose spirit receaueth impediment of passages by these thicke and melancholicke fumes: and thus are the actions of the braine altered by melancholie.

Chap. XXIII.

Howe affections be altered.

TOVCHING their affections of feare and sadnesse, sufficiently hath bene sayd before; sauing whether is first in place, and possesseth first the melancholicke heart, it may make some question. In mine opinion, feare is the verie ground and roote of that sorowe, which melancholick men are throwne into. For a continuance of feare, which is of daunger to come, so ouerlayeth the heart that it maketh it as nowe present, which is only in expectation; and although the daunger feared be absent, yet the assurednesse thereof in the opinion of a melancholicke braine is alwayes present, which ingendreth a
sorow

OF MELANCHOLIE. 133

sorow alwayes accompanying their feares. They are hardely moued to anger, except a biting and fretting choler be mixed with their melancholie, or the melancholy be of an aduft kind: by reason they be ouer paffionat another way, and haue their partes of groffer fenfe then eafily to be offended, and the heart not ready to be moued, being of a colder and drier nature: or fo affected by the humor, which being once throughly kindled with that paffion, retayneth the heate longer, and is not eafily brought againe into the former temper. Enuious they are, becaufe of their owne falfe conceaued want, whereby their eftate, feeminge in their owne fantafie much worfe then it is, or then the condition of other men, maketh them defire that they fee other to enioy, to better their eftate: this maketh them couetours of getting, though in expence where their humour moueth them with liking, or a voydance of perill, more then prodigall. Ieloufie pricketh them, becaufe they are not contented with any moderation, but thinke all too little for fupply of their want: efpecially if it ftand in fuch matters as import great fupplie, or otherwife they doe earneftly affect: and are in feare leaft communication breede whole difpoffeffion, or make inequall partition. They interprete readilie all to the worfe part, fufpitious leaft it be a matter of farther feare, and not indifferently weighing the cafe, but poyfing it by their fantafticall feare, and doubt at home. Paffionate they be out of meafure, whereto a vehement obiect & of long con-

nuaunce vrgeth them: this causeth them to be amorous, both because it is a pleasure to loue, which mittigateth their inwarde sorowe and timiditie, thinneth their bloud, and dilateth the heart, and a cause to be beloued againe, which of all thinges liketh the melancholie personnes, being the greatest meanes of comfort vnto them: from which all offices of kindenesse, curtesie, and grace do flowe: this affection riseth not vnto them by purenesse of nature, but by the force of that which draweth them vnto the vehemencie of passion, wherein they so oft times exceede, that it bereaueth them for a time (ielousie excepted) of all other affection. If the melancholie be sanguine adust, then may it supply the want in the obiect, and cause an internall amorous disposition, with such dotage, that maketh no discretion where the affection is bestowed: as he that is of a merrie nature will laugh at his conceit, and the angrie man displeased with his owne shadowe. Thus farre of the simple actions of brayne and heart, which are altered in melancholicke personnes, and the manner howe, with reason of their alteration: other actions are in comparison of these mixed: as mourning, rising of vaine feare, or counterfet miserie, solitarinesse, least occasion of griefe be ministred by companie and resort: silence, thorough retraction of spirits by their passion (except it be in mornfull plaintes) to mitigate the sorowe, and stiffenesse of the instrumentes, besides the disorderly feare and heauinesse which
can

cannot either minister, nor take occasion of familiar conference and communication, wholly transporting them to the concocting of their sorrowfull humour: which breedeth in them (the passion more and more increasing) a negligence in their affaires, and dissoluteness, where should be diligence. Of pace, they are for the most part slowe, except perill cause them to hasten; both by reason of their members not so nimble for motion, and the mind occupied with cogitation and studie stayeth the pace: as we finde our selues affected, when any matter of weight entreth into our meditatation. Moreouer they are giuen to weeping sometimes (if the melancholie be sanguine, they exceed in laughter) sighing, sobbing, lamentation, countenance demisse, & lowring, bashfulnesse, and blushing, the reasons whereof and manner how they arise, because it requireth a larger discourse, I will refer them more particularly to be discussed in seuerall Chapters followinge, with Philosophicall causes, or probabilities (at the least) how euerie one of these are wrought, that you be fully instructed in that speculation of melancholie, and the accidents which followe it, as you are (more then I wish, or standeth with your present comfort) exercised in the practise.

Chap. XXIIII.
The causes of teares, and their saltnesse.

Of all the actions of melancholie, or rather of heauinesse and sadnesse, none is so ma-

manifolde and diuerse in partes, as that of weeping. First of all it putteth finger in the eye, and sheadeth teares: then it baseth the countenaunce into the bosome: thirdlie it draweth the cheekes with a kinde of conuulsion on both sides, and turneth the countenaunce into a resemblaunce of girninge, and letteth the browes fall vppon the eye liddes; it bleareth the eyes, and maketh the cheekes redde: it causeth the heade to ake, the nose to runne, & mouth to slauer, the lippes to tremble: interrupteth the speeche, and shaketh the whole chest with sighes, and sobbes: and such are the companions of this sorowful gesture of weeping: of which I will deliuer you the reason one by one, first beginning with teares. All obiects, or cause of perturbation riseth more or lesse grieuous, or acceptable, as it is taken: and although the cause be greate, if it be not apprehended, it moueth no perturbation at all. This causeth some to sorowe, whereat another reioyceth: and other some to lament, which other some beare out with courage, or haue no such sense of: and to exceede in ioye or sorowe, (except reason moderate the affection) where other some keepe mediocritie: by reason of certaine degree of apprehension: yea though reason beare no part in the moderation. Moreouer seeing it is necessarie, that both braine and hart be disposed in a kinde of Sympathie, to shewe foorth the affection, as they be diuerslie disposed, so may the cause of perturbation more or lesse moue and trouble. As if the brayne be

quicker

quicker of conceit, and of more exact discretion then the heart is ready to yeeld his passion, by reason of a more compact & firme temper, then is it not aunswerable to the apprehended hurte or daunger. If it be more dull, then by reason the apprehension entreth not duly into the consideration of the present state, or imminent perill, the affection aunswereth not the cause. If the hart be more tender, then the braine ready: there is feare and heauinesse oft times, either without cause, or more vehement then cause requireth: and thus it fareth in the rest of the perturbations, these three alwayes concurring in the affection: the outwarde mouer or cause, the apprehension of the braine, and the motion of the hart: according to the varietie & diuerse disposition of which three, the perturbations become distinct in kinde, and diuerse in degree. This is necessarie for you to know, for the more playne deliuerie of the causes of the accidentes before mentioned: and first of teares, whose passion is not euerie kinde of griefe, nor anie one kinde alike taken, neither though the griefe be taken alike, and the cause iust & true, yet doeth the partie not alwayes sheade teares, thus affected. First therefore, for the manifestation of this matter of tears we are to search what kinde of thing it is that moueth weeping, then how it is to be receiued to work this effect, and thirdly of what disposition they are when iust occasion is ministred, and the cause be so taken, that readily signifie their inward passion, by that dolorous outward gesture and action. Of such causes as draw vs into perturbatton & passion, that only which moueth griefe and sorrow of hart causeth teares. Such weeping as seemeth to proceed of ioy is of a mixt cause as shall hereafter be declared, and maketh no exception to that vniuersall cause of teares procured by affliction, or greeuance: for elſe we see no man weep but in ſorow: neither do any ſorow, but vpon occaſion or perſwaſion of calamitie, or hurt, either preſent or to come: ſauing thoſe which are melācholick paſſionate, who notwithſtanding fancie vnto themſelues a counterfet occaſion therof without cauſe. This I need not ſtand vpō, becauſe it is euidēt of it ſelfe, and requireth no farther demonſtratiō, the other two being of greater difficulty, & of more diligent conſideration. Touching the firſt of the two latter, how the affection is moued for weeping, I take it neceſſarie, the paſſion be not very extreame, nor of the higheſt degree of ſorow, neither ſo light and gētle that the obiect be contemned. For the firſt: if the perturbation be too extreame, and as it were rauiſheth the conceite, and aſtonieth the heart, then teares being ordinary, and naturall to a kinde of mediocritie of that paſſion, are not affoorded to an extraordinary affection: euen as a ioy ſuddaine and rare taketh away for the preſent, the ſignification of reioycing, and turneth the comforte which ſhould be receiued into an admiration, in ſteade of mirth and cheare: ſo in greate extremity of feare and heauines, ſorow being conuerted into an aſtoniſhment, the ſenſes rauiſhed, and the benūmed therewith, the

teares

OF MELANCHOLIE.   139

teares are dryed vp or stayed, (being effectes of ordinary and of naturall passion,) and others more straunger come in place, as voydaunce of vrine, & ordure. For as cold in a kinde of degree, moueth sense, and the same extreame becommeth and taketh it quite away: and as exceeding brightnes blindeth, or at the least dazeleth the sight aswell as darknes obscureth the obiect: so an occasion of feare being beyond ordinary cōpasse of naturall passion, seemeth to the heart, & vnderstanding of another sort, then whereat to sorow, or teares belong, and the tokens of ordinarie affection are due: which flow not, by reason (through that greate perturbation) nature is wholly violated, and keepeth no course of accustomed order: or becaufe such is the flight of nature, from that which she so abhorreth, that hiding her self in her owne cēter, she draweth with her those humidities, which easily follow with the spirites and blood, and are not seperable for vsuall excretion, besides that contraction of her poores, whereby the effluxe of teares is hindered: this in my opinion is the cause: why extremity of terror or heauines restraineth teares, especially if a fright haue gone before: which is of greatest force to make this perturbation, and to shut vp the poores of our bodies. This appeareth in such as are scarred: whose haire seemeth to stand vpright & stiffe through that contraction. So then the same cause of passion in kind differing by degrees, both dolorous & full of calamity nowe causeth abundance of weeping, & gusheth out into brookes of teares, and anon drieth them al vp, through deſtruction of the minde, and ſtupiditye as it were of the hearte: as though the cauſe of morning were altogether remoued. If you do require example in the ſelfe ſame perſon of weeping, and refraining from teares in the ſame kind of obiect, yet differing in degree, that is moſt ſinguler which is reported by Ariſtotle in the ſecond booke of his rhetoricke, out of Herodotus of Amaſis king of Ægypt. We are moued with compaſſion only (ſayeth he) at the affliction of ſuch familiars, as are not very nighly knitte vnto vs, either by acquaintance or affinitie: and of the calamitie of diuerſe moſt deere friends or allies, we haue not compaſſion: but we are affected with their hurte, as with our owne: wherfore it is reported of Amaſis that although he did not weepe for his ſonne, whome he ſawe led to be put to death: yet at the calamitie of his friende Philippus, he ſhed teares: for that which in his friend was pityfull, ſhewed in his ſonne horrible, and terrible to behold: now terror, chaſeth away, & ſwalloweth vp al cōpaſſion. Which hiſtory of Amaſis, maketh cleere al doubt in this point, and confirmeth that which we propound by the reaſon of one of the moſt grauest philoſophers. As this ouer vehement feare dryeth vp theſe ſpringes of teares, or ſhutteth vp the paſſages that no way is giuen for them to diſtill: ſo the cauſe being light, and not greately vrging the heart, nature vſeth not to make ſuch ſhew of ſorow: ſo that at ſmall matters or ſo taken, no man vſeth to weepe. Children (for want of vnderſtanding) in a manner weepe at all occaſions

of

OF MELANCHOLIE.

of offence alike: which tyme and age afterward correcteth. Thus then in my opinion the affection is to be disposed for weeping: euen in a meane, betwixt that light regard of perill or calamitie wherewith no man is moued to teares, and that vehement extremitie, which ingendreth amazednes and astonishment, wherewith nature either is benummed as it were, and dazeled with the extremitie of passion, and neglecteth her ordinarie signification of sorow, in a case so farre extraordinarie: or else so farre withdraweth her selfe into the center of the bodie with her spirite, blood, and humiditie, and closeth vp her poores so straightly, that neither matter of teares is readie, nor passage free for them to distill by. For the naturall passages and such as depend not vpon voluntarie opening or shutting (as of the bladder, & stoole) so farre only are open, as they be distended and filled with blood, humour, & spirite: which being withdrawen as in a dead bodie, they close together like an empty bagge. But why then (say you) do some make vrine for feare: and why doth not nature withold it, aswell as teares, being a kinde of excremét not much vnlike? The reason is readie: such retention as is performed by muscle & animall faculty, descending from the brayne by sinues, is of another sorte, then that which is accomplished by astriction of poore: againe such excrementes as are already congregated into a place of recept, from whence they are to be voided out of the body hereafter, are not of like códition with that which hath as yet no seperatió

For the first pointe; the bladder, as also the fundament, haue ech of them a certaine round muscle, which hath power of opening and closing within it selfe: which opening, way is giuen to the excrement, that of it selfe (finding passage) issueth out of the bodie: or without opening (and it be a liquid excrement as vrine is) if the muscle shutt not close, or retentiue feebled, it voydeth also, though not so plentifully as being full open. Now in feares that exceede, the spirites influent into that muscle (as al are such that pertaine to sence and motion) are caled backe, as I haue before declared, to their proper fountaines, and so it being left destitute, recciueth a kinde of paraliticall disposition for the time, and sayleth in his office, which is the cause of such vnuoluntary excretion. Now if you consider & remember how the vrine passeth from the kideneys by those lōg vessels, you shall well perceiue there can be no refluxe backward, though it be forced. for they discēd not directly, opening théselues as a touch hole into a gune, but sloplings betwixt the substance of the bladder, with certaine slender and thinne skinnes, which immediatly after the entraunce of the humour close vp, in such sort, as the fuller the bladder is, the firmer is their hold, as you may see in the leather clacke of a paire of bellowes: experience hereof is made manifest in a bladder, which being blowen retaineth the aire and suffereth not to vent, though it haue enterances, such as I haue spoken for the vrine. This then is one hinderaunce why the vrine can not be retracted

the

OF MELANCHOLIE. 143

the way being made vp by those skinnes, & the manner of the entraunce such of that excremēt into the bladder, why such stopping can not be in them, as falleth out by closing of poores, that happeneth to other partes through euacuation for these passages are neither opē, because they be full: nor closse, because they be emptie, but are the one for the other, at our voluntary pleasures: to this is the largenes of the passages to be added, which hinder the close sinking of all sides together, with the position of the body downeward direct: and thus much for the difference of the retention and excretion, and how by reason the partes containing the exerement no calling backe of humors can be, as in other parts which haue fluxe and refluxe free. Touching the manner of excremēt, this difference also is to be holden, that such humours as are not yet seperated for euacuation, follow the course of spirites, and ebbe and flow with them, being within the regiment of nature, which the vrine contained in his naturall vrinall, and attending the opening of the passage and destitute of those actiue spirites can not doe: and this I take to be the causes, why in extreame passions of feare, vrine may passe againſt his wil, that notwithstanding can shed no teares by the same extremity. The third pointe remaineth, for the more easie declaration of this dolefull gesture, of what disposition of body they are of, who are apt to teares. They are almost altogether of a moist, rare, and tender body, especially of brayne and heart, which both being of that temper, carie the rest of the parts into like difpofition: this is the caufe why children are more apt to weepe, then thofe that are of greater yeares, and women more then men, the one hauing by youth the body moift, rare & foft, and the other by fex. Whereby teares both eafily flow, and are fupplied with plentifull matter, if with rarenes of body and humidity, the braine aboue the reft exceede that way: and the eyes be great, & vaynes & paſſages there about large: thẽ wāteth ther nothing to the foũtain of tears, euẽ vpõ fmal occafiõ: cõtrarily they which haue their bodies drier by nature, and more cõpact, and the paſſages and poores clofe, as men in comparifon of women & children: fuch hardly yeeld forth that figne of forrow though the occafion may require it. Thus you vnderftãd what occafion moueth weeping, how taken, and what ftate of bodie they be of, that eafily water their cheekes, when forow and calamitie afflicteth. Now let vs confider the matter of teares, what it is, and whence particularly, and properly they flow, and manner how. The matter is the excrementitious humiditie of the brayne, not contained in the vaynes: for elfe would teares not be cleare, nor of a waterifh colour: but refembling the colour of vrine, receiue a tincture from the thinneft parte of the blood, and fo appeare yellow, except the ftraining of the humour might feeme to clarifie them, which can not fo be. For, ftraining, although it caft away impuritie, it altereth not colour: as ftrayne claret wyne as oftẽ as you will, it keepeth ftil the colour. Againe the tincture of yellow; being of a cholericke whay in

hinder

OF MELANCHOLIE.

the blood which is most thinne, would nothing hinder the passage of the teare, nor remaine behind in the strainer. Then we may resolue vpon this point, that teares rise of the brains, thinnest & most liquide excrement; whereof (being the moystest part of the whole bodie, and twise so much in quantitie as the braine of an oxe) it hath great plenty, euen more then anie other part, both in respect of his temper, and largenesse. This excrement is voyded ordinarily by the palate, the nose, and the eyes, by certaine passages ordained for vaines, arteries, and sinues, from that carnell which is placed in the sadle of the bone called the wedge, which is direct ouer the palate of the mouth: this carnell is there placed, that the excremét might not rush suddenly into these parts, but gently distill into them. The most ordinarie passage of thinne humour is by the pallate and nose: the pallate receaueth it directly, the nose from the eyes; lest they should be molested by continuall fluxe: into the eyes it floweth by the passage of the second couple of nerues, which serue to moue the eye, not entering the substance of them, but passing on all sides floweth to the eyes, and from thence is receaued of the fleshly carnell in the inner corner of the eye, and so passeth into the nose, and voydeth out, to purge the head thereby: and this is the ordinarie course of that humiditie, which voyded from the braine into the nose. Vpó occasió of grief, or trouble of smoke or wind, this thinne liquor floweth fró all partes, & is receaued of another fleshly carnell vnder the

K

vpper eye lid towards the eares, & from thence also watereth them, and trickleth downe the cheekes. So then you perceaue the matter of teares,& by what streames it voydeth, and how it is conueighed: it remaineth last of all to lay open vnto you what causeth the fluxe out of the eyes, seeing ordinarily it should passe into the nose, or through the palate be voyded out at the mouth; and how in weeping, nature dischargeth her selfe of this excrement. For clearing of which point, you must call to remembrance the kinde of passion, wherewith nature is charged in matter of griefe or feare; which is an enforcement of flight into her owne center, not hauing whither else to flee: whereby she gathereth in one her spirits, and bloud, & calleth them in, partly withdrawing them from that fearefull obiect, & partly by vniting of forces, inableth her selfe to make greater resistance against that which annoyeth. These spirites are such as passe from the principall partes, of the heart, braine, and liuer, and giue life, nourishment, sense and motion to the rest of the members of our bodies. So then the braine being thus replenished with his flowing spirites, is fuller then it was before, and of necessitie warmer, heat alwayes accompanying spirit: with the spirite, refloweth also the bloud, and humours: and that all may become safe, nature maketh such contraction of the substaunce of the braine, and partes thereabout, that as one desirous to hold fast with his hand that which is apt to flowe forth, loseth by his hard handlinge and compression, which otherwise he might retaine,

OF MELANCHOLIE.

taine, so it expresseth that which by thinnesse is readie to voide, and forcing with spirit, & pressing with contracted substance, signifieth by shower of teares, what storme tosseth the afflicted hart, and ouercasteth the cheerfull countenaunce. And this is the manner of the watering of the sorowfull cheekes, and visage disfigured with lamentatiō, which being by this double meanes inforced, issue in more plentie, then the passage into the nostrells can readilie discharge: the aboundance whereof drencheth the eyes, & ouerflowing the brimmes of the eye liddes, filleth the bosome with teares. This causeth the nose to runne, and the mouth to slauer: euen the sudden breach of these waters, faster seeking vent, then agreeth with natures ordinarie auoydaunce. They are salt of tast, through that heate of the eye, which turneth easily that excrement into saltnesse, besides the mixture of the salt humiditie which is alwayes about it. For the eye of any one being touched with the tong, giueth a manifest releafe of saltnesse: which riseth of that moyst excrement, altered into such tast by the eyes heate. That the eyes be exceeding in heate, besides manifest experience of of touch, the plenty of spirit which they ordinarily possesse, the store of arteries and vaines, the plenty of fat round about, the celeritie of motion do argue sufficiently the same. Neither is that ordinarie passage of humidity frō the brain, whereby their heate may be tempered, lest they become thereby sore, and withered, the least argument of their hote temper, which is not affor-

K ij

foorded to any part of the bodie the hart onely excepted. Lastly the aptnesse to be offended with heate, and readie offence taken that way, sufficiently declareth whereto their nature bendeth.

Chap. xxv.
Why and howe one weepeth for ioy, and laugheth for griefe: why teares and weeping indure not all the time of the cause: and why the finger is put in the eye.

IN the former chapter mention was made of weeping for ioy: here you may demaund a reason, why a ioyfull passion, yeeldeth forth so sorowfull an action; neither do they that weepe faine, as a man will counterfet laughter: for tears cannot be counterfetted, becaule they rise not of any action or facultie voluntarie, but naturall: & the weeping caused of ioy is as hartie, as that which riseth vpon conceit of sorowe. We do see in the works of nature contrary effects wrought by the same cause; so the same effect ensueth vpon contrary causes, through the diuerse maner of the working. You see how the Sunne altereth the whitenelle of a mans skinne into blacknesse, and how it maketh cloth white, it softeneth waxe, and hardeneth clay. Againe we see howe the cold withereth the herbe, as doth the heate: and causeth the earth to be warme, that the fountains smoke againe, as doth the Sunne: and is as requisite with vs in his season, for the fertilitie of the earth, as the reflexion of the Sunne beames. What maruell then, if contraries in paſsions bring forth like effects; as to weepe & laugh, both for ioy & ſorow? For as it is oft ſeene that a man weepeth for ioy, ſo is not ſtraunge to ſee one laugh for griefe; whereof examples are dayly: as if a man taketh vp that which is burning hote, hauing thought it had bin cold, he will laugh at the hurt he feeleth: likewiſe if one aſſay to handle another mans wound, the woūded will declare the diſcontentment with laughter: euen as a mā that is tickled, will laugh though he take no pleaſure in tickling, but rather miſlike & diſcontentmēt. With ſuch kind of laughter did Democritus grieue at the vanities of this life: which alſo moued Heraclitus to weep. And ſometimes in vrgent diſtreſſe, the anguiſh and vexation of mind, is declared w̄ this kind of Sardoniā laughter, as if the hart toke pleaſure, wherat it is grieued. This is cleare, & needeth no lōger diſcours: the reaſon is not ſo euident, which I will nowe make plaine vnto you. As you heard before how teares in ſorowe do iſſue out of the eyes by compreſſiō, & that internal fulneſſe of ſpirits, & heat which forceth out theſe teares; ſo ioy & gladnes being an enlargement of the hart, & braine, & all the internal parts, eſpecially of the ſpirits, which do as it were iſſue out, to welcome the ioyfull obiect, partly thaough the enlargement of the paſſages, & partly through the acceſſe of ſpirits to the outward parts, the moyſture before mentioned is forced out of the eyes, & diſtilleth into drops of teares: eſpecially if cōmiſeration & cōpaſſiō be mixed therw̄: ſuch was Ioſephs weping ouer his brethrē; framed of ioy of their preſence and compassion of their estate: and so did Ionathan weepe ouer Dauid; and Dauid ioying at Ionathans kindenesse, with commisseration of his teares, exceeded him in weeping. This most commonly falleth out, when he whom we loue hath escaped daunger, or we thinke through ouer longe absence, somewhat vnprosperous might, or hath befallen him. Nowe the consideration of the present safety, mingled with remembrance of perill or want, for the present, breaketh out into teares, which are easily to be voyded, both through compression, as hath bin before shewed, and by forcible expulsion. I see you desire farther, as well why griefe procureth laughter, as strange an effect from the cause, as teares are from ioy & comfort. Before I lay this open vnto you, ye are to knowe what partes are first affected with laughter, and how they drawe others into the same fellowship of action. The parts which first are affected in laughter, are the hart and the midriffe, wherto the hart by his call and skinne is more straightly fastened then in beasts; the obiect of laughter being a ridiculous thing, mixed of pleasure and displeasure (else were it not ridiculous) causeth the hart to moue with great celerity his contrary motions of opening, and shutting, which being so repugnaunt, cause a maruelous agitation in the part, by this agitation, and straight coupling of the heart to the midriffe, which draweth by consent other parts into like motion, the laughter is deliuered by interrupted expiration: by reason the midriffe in his contraction is not suffered quietly to

finish

finish it, but is by the harts trouble restrained &
slowed in his fall. Thus knowing the cause of
laughter, and the instruments of the gesture, I
shall more easily manifest vnto you, why a man
may sometimes laugh for griefe and discontentment, as well as weep for ioy. Of all the muscles
in the bodie, the midriffe is the most noble, and
of greatest vse, whose action is in continual motion, and neuer ceaseth, not so much as in sleep
(when all the rest take their ease) for the necessitie of breathing: with this muscle do accord diuerse others; especially those of the neather iaw
and cheekes and lippes, taking their nerues frō
the fourth couple increased by the sixt, which
rise from the pith of the chine in the necke. So
then, the midriffe being affected with any kinde
of extraordinarie motion (as it is in grief) easily
draweth the cheekes, and lippes into like motiō.
But how is the midriffe affected in griefe? euen
much like as it is in laughter: that is to say, hindred in his free falling by the contraction of the
hart, which in griefe calleth in his spirits, closeth
it selfe, & filleth the neighbour parts with more
store of bloud then is ordinarie; which being so
replenished, the midriffe is drawne with the call
of the hart, and hath not his owne libertie in his
contraction: by which meanes the expiration is
deliuered by fits, and not wholly, as in ordinary
breathing, the midriffe (resembling in vse the
leather of a paire of bellows) being ioyned roūd
about to the sides of the chest: which aunswereth the two boords of the bellowes. This also
draweth the consent of the lippes and cheekes,

K iiij

the muscles thereof agreing with the midriffe in their nerues, which make like contractiō to that in laughter, after a counterfet manner in paine and ache that one presently feeleth or feareth. The other kinde, which is of griefe of minde, as that of Hanniball for the distresse of Carthage, and his present calamitie, is of a mixed cause, compounded of some ioy, which riseth of confidence of remedie or reuenge, which causeth a dilatation of ioy, entermeddled with contractiō of griefe: so a man that hath receaued a displeasure of his enemy, and assured howe he may be euen with him, will laugh, though he haue indignation at the displeasure, vpon hope of requittance: whereof riseth a certaine ioye mixed with griefe, that forceth out a Sardonian, bitter laughter, short, and ouertaken with more griefe, which with vapor and spirit, through that dilatation of the hart, filleth the cheekes, and causeth their muscles to be withdrawne to their heads, shew their teeth, and fashion the countenance into that kind of grinning which is apparant in laughter. Thus much by the way of laugter, by occasion of that weeping, which falleth vnto such as vpon cause of ioy breake out into teares. If you desire to knowe more of this merie gesture, I referre you to a treatise of laughter, written by Laurence Ioubert of Mountpellier, a Philosopher, and Phisitian, in my iudgement not inferiour to any of this age. The cause why weeping endureth not all the time of the sorow, but most commonly at the first brunt onely of griefe tears are shed, is partly by reason time acquainteth

teth the hart with the sorowe, so is the contraction lesse, the daunger not being so straunge. Againe, that moysture is partly emptied, which ministreth matter vnto teares, & reason in time dealeth with the affection, which peraduenture moderateth the griefe, whereby it lesse vrgeth. The finger is vsually put in the eye in weeping, by reason the teare falling into the eye with his saltnesse procureth a kind of itching about the carnell of teares, which requireth ayde of the finger to be expressed at their first fal: afterward the part acquainted with that qualitie, and one teare drawing on another, such expression is not so necessarie. Besides this cause of rubbing the weeping eye, a strange matter therin requireth wyping, which also moueth the finger to hast to the eye watered with teares: but this is after a while; the other before almost anie teare fall, as though they were expressed with rubbing. And thus much touching the causes of teares, which beare the greatest part in weeping: nowe ye shall vnderstand howe other partes of that gesture are perfourmed, and by what meanes.

Chap. XXVI.

Of other partes of weeping: why the countenance is cast downe, the forehead loureth, the nose droppeth, the lippe trembleth, the cheekes are drawn, and the speech is interrupted.

IN weeping the countenance is cast downe, by reason the spirits are retracted, which are the authors (by tonicall motion) of erection: as a maste corded on all sides standeth erect: which in sorow being withdrawē from the muscle, causeth them to yeeld to the poyse of the head: and so bendeth it downeward, wherto it is more enclined then backeward: by reason the rowells of the neckbone, with their snaggs hinder that inclination. The forehead lowreth after a paraliticall fashion, being destitute of his spirites, and all the former partes filled with that excrementitious moisture of teares before mentioned: which is in that aboundance in persons moist of braine, tender and rare of poores, that not finding sufficiēt way at the eyes, it passeth through the nose, as the other part by the palate, into the mouth, and so filleth all full of teares and slauer. The lipe trembleth, becaufe the spirite which should vphold it in his right position, is now in greatest measure departed: so that the waight of the lippe, striuing with the imbecillitie of the parte, causeth a trembling, which is betwixt erection, and plaine declination: as if a man hold a thing too heauy till he beginne to be weary: though at the first he hold it steady, at the lēgth striuing aboue his power to beare it, maketh his hand to quake and tremble, the remnaunte of strength, striuing with the weight. The vpper lippe remaineth steadie and still, becaufe it hangeth, and requireth no proppe of erection: yet appeareth it somewhat longer then before, being fully stretched out with the weight, and not borne vp, & restrained by the spirit. The cheeks are drawen much like as in laughter: not by any

influence

influence of the liuely spirite, which in laughter replenisheth the countenance, and causeth the eyes to sparcle, and filling the muscles of the cheekes with a subtle vapour, causeth them to strayne for the auoydance: as in streaking, the muscles are contracted to exclude a vaporous excrement: but the contraction of the cheekes in weeping seemeth to me, not to rise of any other cause, then by an excrementitious vapour, which passeth with the humiditie of teares, frō the braine into the cheekes, and forceth nature to make contraction to discharge it selfe of that vapour: ioyned with the cōsent, which is betwixt the muscles of the iawes and lipps with the midriffe: whose remission, and slackening, being hastened by the contraction of the harte in griefe, contracteth also the foresaid lipps and cheekes, with which it consenteth by the fourth and sixt paire of nerues, deriued into both partes, from the marow of the chine bone of the neck. These are also the causes, of the whole deformitie of the face in weeping, which chiefely contracteth the visage in expiration, in which the heart hath more power ouer the mydriffe being slakened, then in inspiration, wherein by dilating of the chest for vse of breath it is extēded. The speach is interrupted in weeping, becauſe the chest in expiration doth not fall and sinck, by gentle declination equally: but hindred by that contraction of the heart, remitteth his extension, as it were by stroakes: as if a man would take a paire of bellowes, and not suffer them being enlarged, and full of aire to shutt of themselues, but by an vnequall pressing of the handes, cause them to puffe by fittes, and part the blowing into sundry blastes, which at once might be auoyded. So the voyce rising of the ayre expired, as that is voyded, in like sort the voyce is fraimed: which causeth those that weepe to speake more indistinctly, and diuided sentences, then when they are free from that affection. Moreouer speach doth require not onely the yeeldinge of the chest through the poyse, but standeth in neede also of the intercostall muscles, and those of the top of the windpipe with thē of the bely which throgh griefe or feare being now not so replenished with spirites, the authors of motion of those muscles, can not deliuer the voyce smoth and vniforme as before, more then a childe is able sufficiently to way downe by his strength of hand a smithes bellow, that is forced by poyces to finish that which strēgth would perform at once. Neither is the speach interrupted, and broken only by the disorderly expiratiō, but the inspiratiō being by sobs cutteth also the voyce, & marreth the distinct pronūtiatiō, the cause whereof as also of sighing I will deliuer vnto you in the next chapter. Thus you haue (sobbing excepted) the reasons of all the partes of weeping, so farre as my coniecture by reason in matters so hidden can gather: I will proceede to the causes of sighing and sobbing, and how they be procured, and by what meanes, and so finish the whole mournefull gesture of weeping.

CHAP.

Of Melancholie.

Chap. XXVII.
The causes of sobbing and sighing and how weeping easeth the heart.

Besides the former actiōs of sorow, weping is for the most part accompanied (if it be vehement) with sobbes and sighes: of which two, sobbing is neuer without weeping, sighes are ordinarie and common vppon causes that force no teares, as euery one hath experiēce. For vnderstanding of the causes of sobbes, it is necessarie for you to call to minde that which hath bin said of the vse of the Diaphragma, or midriffe, and the outward intercostalls, or outward muscles betwixt the ribbes, and the manner how the hearte is affected in griefe and sorrowe. The dilating of Diaphragma is to enlarge the chest for taking breath. This is onely required, if we be not more thē ordinarilie vrged to breath: which if we be, then doe the outwarde muscles of the ribbes dilate the chest also, and so encrease the inlargement. Now when matter of griefe inforceth teares, the Diaphragme, and the muscles recciue a weakenes, by reason of retraction of spirites, that they are faine for the dilatation of the chest to make mo pulls then one, as you heard before in the motion of contraction, so that the breath is not drawen at one straining of their coares and fibers, but by diuers inspiration: besides the heat of those partes being retracted, maketh them lesse plyable vnto the force of the muscles: whereby the respiration is with more difficultie perfoormed, which requireth more vse of dilatation, then before: by reason the heate about the heart it selfe is now greater then before the passion, which bringeth thereto a kind of suffocation. That cooling of the heart which is sensibly felt by suddaine euill tydinges, or mishappe vnlooked for, or whatsoeuer new calamitie, riseth through accesse of the blood and spirits: which although they be hote, yet wanting somewhat of that heate which is feruét, and naturall to the heart, and of the heat of those spirites which are resident there, for the time seemeth to coole in comparison of the heat which the heart felt before: as a mā would cast hote water to that which boyleth most feruently: which although it be hote, yet inferiour in degree to the heate of feruentnes, it mitigateth the scalding heate, and slaketh the boyling. In like manner at the first recourse of these humours, and raunging spirites, although the heart seeme to receiue a chilling, yet anone by contraction, and plenty of spirites which are apt to take heat it receiueth a greater necessitie of breathing, which being not aunswered through imbecillitie of the breathing parts, dischargeth the office of respiration by sobbes, which should be performed by one draught of breath. And these I take to be the causes of sobbing. Sighing hath no other cause of mouing then to coole and refresh the hearte, with fresh breath, and pure aire, which is the nourishment and foode of the vitall spirites, besides the cooling which the heart it selfe receiueth thereby. The heart being contracted as hath bene said, deliuereth not so freely his ly his sootie and smokie excrementes, whereby the spirites become impure, and it boyleth with more distemper:which necessitie of fresh spirite and coole ayre enforceth a deeper enlargement of the chest then is ordinarie;in which not only the midriffe playeth his parte, but outward intercostalls or middle muscles of the ribbes, besides certaine of the shoulders, doe their indeuour to this so necessary an office. Moreouer it is very probable that the midriffe by accesse of humours and vapours to the partes there about is charged with vaperous superfluitie, which is by stretching it selfe, as in yawning, auoyded: when the muscles are distended by any vapour, of what sort soeuer it be of, being plentifull and aboundant, it stirreth them to a contraction, which causeth a kinde of pressing, wherby they deliuer themselues of this excrement. This in yawning causeth that gaping, & sometimes accompanied with streaking, when we finde our selues vnlustie, and vndisposed to stirre or exercise: which falling to the midriffe, may cause a kinde of sighing,when a man hath no cause: as hauing cause,it helpeth it foreward.For whosoeuer yawneth, shall perceiue his chest and midriffe dilated in such manner as in sighing,&feele about the heart a kinde of refreshing: euen as when he sigheth. To these causes may be added the weight of the hart, which is by reason of the accesse of humours about his vaynes and arteries to his contraction,increased:whereby it lyeth more heauily vpon the midriffe then before the burthen whereof it seeketh to ease it self of, by such streitching, which somewhat lifteth vp the hearte for the time, and so the Diaphragma is recōforted: so that the necessity of fresh aire, the cooling of the hearte, the easing of the burthen therof vpō the midriffe, the auoiding of vaporous excrements out of the midriffe, seeme to me causes final, & the midriffes dilatatiō, whose motion the whole chest followeth the efficient cause of sobing & sighing. And thus much cōcerning the two dolorous actions of sighing & sobbing, whereto after I haue added how it easeth the heart to weepe & sobbe, I will end this chapter. By reason of the withdrawing of the blood & spirites about the heart in feare, and sorow, it is necessary, that much vapour should arise, stirred vp by the heat therof working vpō the moisture these vapours besides the ordinarie excrements of the brayne before mentioned, may yeeld another parte vnto teares, being congeled in the brayne, and vpper partes that are thicke, coole, membranous, inclosed with the skull, and placed ouer the rest, as a stillitorie helme ouer the bodie. Now weeping by making auoydāce to these vapours, doth discharge that fulnes wherewith it was before strayned and oppressed. These vapours cause that rednes in the cheekes, and about the eares of those that weepe, heateth the face, and causeth the head to ake, whereof the heart being eased, receiueth a farther enlargement then at the beginning of the griefe, and so enioyeth that small comfort which weeping affoordeth. It may seeme probable that the sobbing and sighing (differing onely in that sobbes large are sighinges interrupted, and sighes sobbes at large) if they be not vehement and long by agitation of the chest expelling of the smothered vapours, and drawing in of fresh aire, geue also some comfort: if they be vehement, then shake they the hart and midriffe too much, and cause a sorenesse about those partes, especially about the hart spoone, which is most trauelled in sobbing, and whereto the midriffe is fastened. Thus much concerning those actions which are animall, and ly in our power (some absolutely, and some after a sort) to do or not to do, altered by passion of sorowe, and falling into melancholie persons: it resteth to shewe, howe melancholie procureth this laughing and weeping, and so to proceede to those naturall actions which are altred by this humour, with the reason of such effects.

Chap. XXVIII.

Howe melancholie causeth both weeping and laughing, and the reasons how.

IT hath bene before declared how melancholy causeth feare and sorowe of hart, by false imagination, raised through fearefull vapours rising to the braine, and passing by the hart, euen before the imagination be moued, causeth a contraction thereof: which is the action of feare: this feare breedeth sorowe; the sorow and feare accompanying ech other, make such contractiō as before hath bene sayde to be cause of teares;

the matter being partly supplied by the ordinary excrements of the braine, and partly through those vapours which arise from the hart ouercharged with concourse of humours, which are retracted by the spirites; who vpon matter of discontentment haft vnto the place of defence, and assemble together, flying the irksome obiect, and addressing them selues as it were to make resistance. The partes about the eyes being porous and rare, the braine moyst, and the partie apt to weepe, vpon this melancholie disposition springeth that issue of teares out of melancholicke eyes: and these I suppose to be the causes, why melancholicke persons without anie outward occasion, fall into weeping and lamentation. Why they laugh, and that excessiuely, the cause is of more difficultie to finde out, and the reason not so manifest, whereof as I am ledde by coniecture and probabilities, I will deliuer you mine opinion. You may remember how the midriffe next vnto the hart is the chiefe cause of laughter; so that of necessitie one of these must be affected in that action. The heart is alwayes affected in true laughter, and not alwayes in a fained kind, which is only a shaking of the chest, and retraction of the lippes, without the liuely and chearfull eye, fraught with the ioyfull spirites, which replenish the merie countenaunce. This kinde is that which melancholicke persons without obiect breake out into; except the melancholie rise of adustion of bloud, and become blacke choller, which affecteth also the heart with a faigned conceit of merinesse; euen

Of Melancholie.

as wine giueth it comfort, and ſtirreth the ſpirits to that liuelines & cheare, wherof euery one hath experience. Nowe then for the better laying open this melancholick action, we are to diſtinguiſh of laughter: wherof there be two ſorts; the one is true and vnfaigned, riſing from a comfort and reioycing of the hart; and the other a counterfet and falſe, wherein the heart receaueth no contentment, but either it ſelfe, or the midriffe moued diſſorderly with ſhaking by anie annoyance; and moueth alſo the cheſt, and muſcles of the iawes and cheekes by conſent of nerues, and ſo counterfetting a laughinge geſture, wherein the heart taketh no pleaſure. The former kinde may riſe of inward cauſe, as well as outward; when the vapour of aduſt melancholie of bloud, or rather when it firſt taketh that heate, perfumeth the heart with a pure & cleare fume, whereat it is allured to ioye and cheare: which vapour and fume riſinge of the moſt mildeſt and temperate humour, before the full aduſtion be accompliſhed, and mixed with the other humours and ſpirites, breedeth that pleaſaunt vaine, which ouertaketh melancholicke perſons, which peraduenture otherwiſe not ſo delayed, would turne the heart to annoyance. This way melancholie carrying a winie and aromaticall ſpirit, raiſed by that heat, may procure an harty laughter, & not only diſpoſe as wine doth, the ſpirit thus rayſed being more familiar thē that of wine, & ſo compelling as it were the hart to breāk forth into that actiō of reioycing. The falſe kinde of laughter which

L ij

proceedeth firſt from the midriffe, moſt commonly is affected by melancholie, through a tickling vapor or ſpirite, which riſeth frō the lower parts, and ſtirreth the midriffe; as they which are woūded in the cheſt, and vpon dreſſing are there about touched, do plainly perceaue to moue, & ſhake, and retract it ſelfe, (whoſe motion the cheſt followeth) and to force out a counterfet manner of laughter, whereof the hart hath no part; nor countenance, ſauing the girning of the mouth, which is here but ſmall, maketh anie pleaſant ſhew. This accident pertaineth chiefly to that melancholie which reſteth about the ſplene, the meſaraicke vaines, and port vayne of the liuer; which breatheth an itching and tickling breath, whereof the midriffe takinge the ſence, ſhaketh & moueth, with indeuour to ſhun the vnwelcome gheſt, and to auoyde the touch thereof. Now that being once moued, the other inſtruments of laughter aunſwere with like motion, and all agree in this counterfet geſture, which in appearance ſeemeth like the pleaſaunt looke of a light and merily diſpoſed hart. This accident of laughter for the moſt part is whē the melancholy paſſion beginneth, or anon after, before the bloud getteth a ferther egerneſſe, and thoſe iolie ſpirites be waſted: which after they once be ſpent, & the heat either outragious, or delayed or diſtinguiſhed by vnaptnes of matter, thē is the comedy turned into tragedy, pleaſantnes into fury, & in the end, mirth into mourning much like as it fareth with ſuch as intemperatly take in their cups, & are ouer ſurfeted with wine

or

or strong drink; these of them that are of nature cold and dry, & of this melancholie complexion voyd of adustion, at the first cup receaue a maruelous cheering about the hart, the drinesse and coldnesse of their inward parts being soked and steeped as it were, like dry leather in oyle: if they proceed farther, the former modestie anon altereth it selfe into the contrarie extremitie of chat and excessiue babling, the spirit of the wine ouerruling the spirit of their natural complexion: yet a litle more sipping, and this melancholy receaueth such heat, as rage and furie entreth possession of hart, and braine; and as he had taken a draught of Circes cup, he fareth in respect of maners & behauiour, as though he were turned into a wild beast. In the end with farther carouses of excesse, the wine, for the while quite dispossessing the spirits of their regiment & office, and quenching as it were the one heate, & delaying the naturall heat of his body with immoderate quātity, the mirth & chere, the pleasant talk, the rage & furie giue place, & in steed of that iolitie, succedeth silence, stupiditie, sleep & sottishnesse. So in melācholie, while that drie & subtile spirit is supplied with conueniēt matter, & is lightned in the melancholick part, all is on the hoigh for a time, which being consumed by heat, the store therof being but small in respect of the grosse residēce, the melancholick person becometh afterward sad, heauy, & vncherful. Thus you perceiue (I think) sufficiently how melancholick persons, some laugh & some weepe, & in the same melancholicke, what causeth mirth, & what teares. Before I proceede to the naturall actions chaunged and depraued by melancholy, I cannot passe ouer an action which is verie vsuall to melancholicke folke, and that is blushing, with shunning of the looke and countenaunce of men, which the Grecians call Dysopia; and because it requireth a larger discourse then the ende of this Chapter will suffer, I will treate of them in the next.

Chap. xxix.

The causes of blushing and bashfulnesse, and why melancholicke persons are giuen thereunto.

THE affection that moueth blushinge is shame, howsoeuer it riseth, either vppon false conceit, or deserued cause. Shame is an affection of griefe, mixed with anger against our selues, rising of the conscience of some knowne, or supposed to be knowne offence, either in doing that, which ought not to be done, or omitting that which was requisite of vs to be done. This description I will vnfold vnto you more at large: that in shame euery one is grieued, experience maketh plaine, besides reason leadeth thereunto. Euerie passion of the heart is with ioye, or with griefe, either sincere and simple, or mixed, as in ridiculous occasions: in shame there is no absolute ioye nor comfort, therefore there must needs be a displeasantnesse or else a mixt disposition of sorowe and cheare: this there is not, by reason shame casteth downe

the

the countenance, filleth the eye with sorow, and as much as may be withdraweth the liuely and comfortable spirit into the center of the bodie, not vnlike vnto feare and sadnesse. It appeareth mixed with anger, by reason euerie one feeleth a kinde of indignation within him selfe, and offereth as it were a vehement inablinge of him selfe: for the offence wee are angrie with our selues, because the fault is ours, and from vs riseth the cause of griefe; as in absolute anger the cause is from other, and vpon others we seeke the reuenge. Where there is no conscience, there can not be any sense of fault: for that it is which layeth our actions to the rule, and concludeth them good or bad: so although the fault be committed in deede, and yet no conscience made thereof, it is taken for no offence, neither can giue cause of this internall grief & reuengement. To these clauses I ad an offence knowne, or so supposed: for otherwise, though a man be grieued and sorie therefore, yet before it be knowne to others is he not ashamed. This causeth that men make no doubt of doing that in secret, which for shame they would not do openly; yea in such thinges as of them selues are not dishonest, nor disalowable. Moreouer, it ri'eth vpon offence, committed in that thing which lay in our power (as we tooke it) to remedie, or better to haue discharged our selues in doing or omitting. Therefore no man is ashamed of an ague, or of the goute, or to haue broken his legges, or anie such occasion, as to haue bene spoyled, or to die &c. but onely in those thinges wherein we take our selues to haue our part, and to rise vpon our owne default: so are we both ashamed of the action, and of all tokens thereof. Nowe seing that all offence, is neither in doing amisse, or neglecting that should be done, in either of both consisteth matter of shame. The description of shame thus being declared, I proceede to shewe howe it forceth rednesse into the eares and cheekes, and causeth vs neither to beare other mens countenaunces and lookes, nor with courage and boldnesse to beare vp our owne. The griefe that nature conceaueth from our selues, is not so straunge, as that which is foraine, and outward, but farre more familiar, and thence therefore in all partes more known. Moreouer the cause is more transitorie and fading; especially, if the offence be small and of no great note. Againe the griefe is not for anie depriuation of that, whereof the vse is so necessarie, as losse of friendes, goodes, perill, pouertie do all import, nor of anie singular pleasure, wherein nature or will tooke their chiefe contentment. These qualities of shame ioyned with anger, procureth that rednesse in the face, which we call blushing. The tincture of redde ariseth on this sort: the heart discontented with the opennesse of the offence, maketh a retraction of bloud, and spirit at the first, as in feare and griefe; and because it feeleth no greater hurt then of laughter, or rebuke of worde, or such like touch, seeketh no farther escape, then a small withdrawing of the spirite and bloud by the first entrance of the perturbation: so that

the

Of Melancholie. 169

the necessitie being no more vrgent, the bloud and spirit breake forth againe more vehemently, and fill the partes about the face more then before, and causeth the rednesse. This is helped forwarde with that anger, which is mixed with shame, which forceth in some sorte, these retracted spirites and bloud to reflowe with more strength, as we see the bloud soone vp of a cholericke person. The passion is not so vehement to close vp the spirits, and to retaine anie longer time, for the cause before alledged; and although it were, yet would the anger, and inwarde reuengement make way to the bloud and spirites, to geue that shamefast colour. Thus you vnderstand what maner of perturbation causeth blushing, what it is, and how it breedeth the staine: but you wil peraduenture say, why do not all that are ashamed blush, and why some more then other some? This I suppose to be cause: in blushing these pointes are to be considered for answer of this question; the qualitie of the bloud and spirit, the passage, & nature or substāce of the face, which receiueth this reflux. If the blud be grosse and thicke, and the passages not so free, then is the course of bloud slow, & the coutenance little altered. If the skin be ouer thick, or ouer rare, thē doth it not admit throgh the thicknes of the spirites, or at the least maketh not that shew, nor retaineth them through the rarenes and thinnes, and by exoperation make no apparaunce of rednes: this is the cause why many ashamed be not so ready to blush. Besides this disposition of spirite, humour and substance of the face, the

measure of the shame more or lesse, helpeth and hindereth blushing. For some there are affected more vehemently, and othersome moderately, & othersome not a whit: who blush not, because they are not at all ashamed. By that hath bin declared you may gather, why the yonger sort, and women easily blush: euen through rarenes of their body and spirites, ioyned with simplicitie, which causeth doubt of offence: and this is the cause why we commend blushers, because it declareth a tender heart, and easily moued with remorse of that which is done amisse, & a feare to offend, and a care least it should cōmit ought worthy of blame. Furthermore it sheweth a conscience quicke, and tender, and an vpright sentence of the minde, agreeable to this ingrauen maximes of good and euill: and thus much shall suffice you for blushing. As for the shunning of mens countenances, and bashfulnes, either in beholding, or being beheld, it riseth vpon a giltines in conceite, or in effect, in that we feare is knowen to others wherein we haue offended, or stand in doubt we shall offend. This conceit causeth vs to hide our selues, and to withdraw our presence from the society of me, whom we feare doe view our faultes in beholding vs, and wherof our presence stirreth vp the remembraunce. Wherefore we being desirous to couer and hyde our offence, seeke also to be hidde and couered, who haue deserued the blame: especially from such of whome we haue greatest reuerence, and of whose estimation and censure we stand most in awe of. Now because the vewing of another
causeth

OF MELANCHOLIE.

causeth the like from him againe, therfore doth the guilty minde abstaine ther from: that it prouoke not the eye of another whome he doth behold: especially if the other party looke vpõ him againe, then is he presently outcountenanced through the guiltie conceite, and ielousie of the crime which he suspect to be reueiled. Moreouer the countenance being as it were the grauen character of the mind, the guilty person feareth least that be red in his forehead, whereof he is guilty in his heart: which augmenteth the griefe, when he seeth himselfe eyed more then (by turning aside his owne countenance) when he beholdeth it not. Thus much touching the former bashfull actions, whether they rise vpon cause, or opinion only: it remaineth of this chapter to shew, how melancholicke persons are much subiect to both, though they haue committed nothing deseruing rebuke, or worthy of shame. That which befalleth youth, by their tender age in blushing, the same in a manner happeneth to melancholicke persons by their complexion: youth and children, if they come in place of reuerend persons will easily blush, not of any fault committed, but of reuerence to the parties: nature as it were secretly in respect, condemning her imperfections in that age, whereof the presence of both maketh a kinde of comparison. Moreouer the nature carefull of that which is seemely and decent, not acquainted with such presence, doubteth of error and vncomelinesse, and distrusting it selfe, blusheth as if offence had bene committed. This is the cause why the yong take occasion sooner then the aged, and why reuerend and vnacquainted presence causeth this passion. They which are of mo yeares, by reason of experience and further knowledge, which breedeth an assurance, more hardly blush, and familiarity and custome maketh greater boldnes. Euen so the melancholick person, through his internall mislike, and cause of discouragement, hath litle assurance or contentment in his actions whatsoeuer: Whereby without cause he easily groweth into a conceite of some absurdity committed where none is: this causeth him to blush, and to expresse by outward rednes of colour the internall passion: especially this befalleth him, if he carrie any conscience of former vice committed: then doth that ouercharge and set all out of order, chiefely if it mingle the passion with feare, and the quality of the blood and spirite, largenes of poores, and disposition of the skinne in the face aunswere thereunto. But how, will you say, can the melancholy person haue his spirite and blood so disposed, which I haue declared to be grosse and thicke, and the passages of their bodies not free? Trueth it is that all melancholicke persons are not so disposed to this action of blushing, by reason they are of blood, spirite, and body vnapt thereunto: but certaine only who haue melancholy not equally disposed, but resteth vnder the ribbes, & anoieth chiefly with his vapour, and who are such not from their parents, but by some accident of diet or euill custome, which notwithstanding retaine as yet the same disposition of their firme

partes

partes they had before : or haue some other humour of thinner substāce, wherby their blood is not so dull of ebbing & flowing: these I take to be the melancholick blushers only, and the rest in all respects farre remoued there from: whose swartnes of the skinne with other impediments both hindereth the recourse of the blood: and if they did blush, ouershadoweth the colour. The same cause which stirreth blushing in melancholicke men, forceth them to auoide assemblies, and publike theaters: and this is common to all melancholickes, howsoeuer they be tempered in their bodies: euen the opinion and fancy of some disgrace from others, who are greatly displeased with themselues, and by their erronious conceite preuent the sentence of others vpon themselues, and condemne that vniustly, which ducly wayed, and without passion, hath no desert of blame. Thus much for these actions of blushing, and bashfullnes.

Chap. xxx.

Of the naturall actions altered by melancholy.

Hitherto you haue had declared the alteration of such actions as lie in our power, & are for the most part arbitrarie: it followeth to shew vnto you the rest which are natural, & are not at our becke, but are performed by a certaine instinct of nature wil we, nil we. These actiōs are of appetite, or of nourishmēt: the actiōs of appetite are of meate and drinke, or of procreation. Touching appetite of meate, melancholy persons haue it for the most part exceeding, and farre surpassing their digesture. The cause why, it is through an aboundance of melancholy, which easily passeth from the splene, the sincke of that humour, to the stomach, whose sowernes prouoketh an appetite of nourishment, to delay that sharpnes which molesteth the mouth thereof: & that you may with more facility conceiue this pointe, marke what I shall say of the splene, the stomach, and the passage of that humour thereinto. The splene lieth vnder the short ribbes on the left side of the stomach backward, and is ordained to purge the blood of melancholick iuice, which it draweth vnto it selfby meane of vaines, and being satisfied with some parte wherewith it is nourished, the remnaunte sower of taste, and as a naturall sawce, it belcheth as it were into the stomach, whose sharpnes causeth a kinde of griefe and knawing therein, especially about the entrance, which is most sensible, & so prouoketh the appetite of nourishment: by whose sweete and familiar iuice, the sharpnes or sowernes of the other is dulled and tempered, & so the byting eased. Besides this sence which the quallity of melancholy offereth to the stomach it (according to the nature of all thinges of that taste) bindeth and contracteth the stomach: which may also be another cause of the encrease of that paine which inforceth to seek after nourishment. Thus then the stomach being subiect vnto the splenetick humour, as it exceedeth or

OF MELANCHOLIE. 175

is more sowre, so doth this appetite more increase. Now in persons melancholicke, the superfluity of this humor is in great abcundance, which thereby the more forceth the appetite: and this I take to be one cause of that greedy hunger, which is more insatiable in melancholicke men then in others. To this may be added the desire that nature hath to seeke and supply, that thicke, grosse and dry humour, with new & fresh nourishment, and to temper the foggy spirites of that humour, with more cleare, fresh and new: these wants of nature happely are another cause of that greedy appetite of melancholicke persons. Their concoction and digestion is not aunswerable to the appetite: through the coldnes of the stomach, both by the melancholicke blood, wherewith it is fedded, and more neighbourhood of the splene, which is a part inclyning from mediocrity to coldnes in temper: this hindereth the concoction. The digestion or distribution faileth through difficulty of passage, both by thicknes and slownes of the melancholy iuice, and narrownes of the way, especially if the partie be by nature, and not through other occasion melancholicke. To this may be added the dulnes of attractiue power of the parts, caused by coldnes and drinesse, and the vnsauorie iuice, in comparison of the pure blood, whereof nature is not pricked so vehemently with the desire. These I take to be reasons of the quicke appetite of melancholicke persons, and slow digestion, and concoction, which partes of the former diuision belonging to nourishment, by order should afterward be handled: but because the comparison with the appetite ministred occasion, you shall take them in this place, and not looke for them hereafter. Whatsoeuer other imbecillity of naturall action about nourishment is depraued by melancholy, the reason may be drawne from that hath bin shewed of the other. They are not so desirous of drinke, although melancholy be a dry humour, both because their coldnes slakeneth the thirst, and their stomacks be moist by want of digestion, which sendeth vp waterie vapours into the mouth, besides the ascent of the humour it selfe, which satisfieth the drought if any be, and preuenteth the desire of drincke. Their stomach is cold through melancholy, which by the aboundance which floweth therein from the splene is cooled, as also by the vicinetie of the same; which lyeth close therunto. The other appetite is of procreation, wherewith or the most parte melancholy persons are more vehemently stirred: the cause whereof I take to be double: the one from the affection of loue, wherewith they are soone ouertaken: the other a windy disposition of their bodies, which procureth that desire. They are allured to loue more easily, because they more admire other then themselues, and being cast downe with cõceite of their owne imperfection, extoll in their fancy that which hath any small grace of louelines in another. The other reason I referre you to reade at large of in treatises of philosophie, writté of the matter in other languages: the grauity and modesty of our tounge not fitting with

phrase

OF MELANCHOLIE. 179

phrase to deliuer such problemes. Thus much shall suffice for the appetite depraued by melancholie: other sorts of naturall actions besides concoction and distribution, (which haue bene before sufficiently to the purpose in hande intreated of) are the retention ouer fast, and assimulation, or turning of the nourishment into our substances imperfect. The first fault riseth chiefly of the drinesse of the parts, which thereby retaine anie humiditie, the slownesse of the humour which maketh no way though nature expell; and if it be an excrement that should passe, the grossenesse wherewith she hath bene acquainted, causeth the offence thereof lesse to be felt, and so nature becommeth more sluttish in cleansing the bodie of his impurities. Againe the sense of such persons is not verie quicke, neither carrieth the excrement anie prickinge of prouocation, which should put nature in remembraunce of auoydance, except immoderate quantitie serue that turne, whereof the drinesse of melancholicke natures is an impediment. The assimilation is faultie by reason of colde; this causeth that morphewe, which ofte staineth melancholicke bodies, and bespeckleth their skinne here and there with blacke staines of this humour: & then the nourishment in steed of supplying the perpetuall fluxe of our bodies, and aunswering in like substance, is (by fault of the parte of melancholicke disposition) depraued, and turned into like iuyce, wherewith the parte is dyed into that blacke coloure. The colour is blacke of the nature of of the humor, and disposition of the part which by imbecillitie is not able to alter it into whitenesse, to the similitude of it self. Hitherto I haue declared vnto you what actions melancholy depraueth; whether voluntary, or naturall; of voluntary, whether of sense and motion, or of affection and perturbation; of naturall whether action of appetite, or belonging to the working of nourishment: of appetite, whether of victualles, or of lust: touching dressing and preparation of nourishment, whether it be coction, digestion, attraction, retention, assimulation or expulsion: it remaineth to deliuer vnto you, what workes are depraued by this humour, and howe it corrupteth the perfection of them.

Chap. xxxi.
How melancholie altereth naturall works of the bodie, iuyce and excrements.

AL the works which rise of naturall actions in our bodies may be reduced to two sorts: the one is naturall iuyce, apt for nourishmēt & building vp the decay of our bodies through the businesse of this life and the internall fire, which continually craueth fuell of victuall: the other is a superfluity which riseth of the masse of meats and drinkes, separated from the pure and nutritiue, by the triall of our naturall heate: as we see the drosse and impuritie of metalles discouered by the fire. This superfluitie nature expelleth out of the bodie, not being of that sinceritie and familiar qualitie, which nourishment is indued

Of Melancholie.

dued with. Both these are altered by this melancholicke disposition, whereof my discourse runneth. The nourishing iuyce (by melancholie) of such nourishmentes as are pure and good receaueth imperfection, and becommeth grosser, thicker, and more crude then by the qualitie of the substance it might be: the rather also, because melancholicke appetite is not proportionall to their digestion, but exceedeth. These causes procure the nourishing iuyce thicke, grosse, and crude, because the heate of melancholicke persons is abated by this humour; which heat is the worker of separation, and maketh subtile & liquide that which of nature hath no contrarie disposition. This nourishing iuyce is either primitiue, and the first whereof the other take beginning and matter; or else deriuatiue and rising frō the primitiue. The primitiue is that which is wrought in the stomach, and is in colour white, liquide, equall, of a cremy substance: in this, as yet, no separatiō is made of place, but wholsome and vnwholsome, excrement and nourishment are mixt together; onely there they are as it were dissolued and broken, and by our heate made more familiar vnto vs, and prepared for other parts more easie handling This is the grosser, for causes before alleaged, and yeeldeth the excrement voyded by stoole, the thickest and grossest of all the rest; which being increased in those qualities by the melancholicke disposition, molesteth them with costiuenesse, and hardnesse of bellie. For through the qualities before mentioned it passeth not so easilie the guts, which besides the foulds they haue, lest we should be oftener then were meet forced to the stoole, they haue plaits ouerthwart, as is to be seene in the inwardes of beasts, which the drie excrement more hardly passeth ouer. Againe, such as are enclined to one excesse of humour, are for the most part lesse prone to another: especially if it hath any contrarie qualitie: so melancholie, exceeding through the cooling of the temper, therewith lesse plenty of choller is engendred; which choler nature serueth her selfe of for a naturall clyster of the intrailes and guts, both to scoure them, and with bitternesse to stir vp more readily the naturall excretion. Of this humour then melancholicke persons possessing but small portion, and the excrement of it selfe grosse & dry, stayeth longer in the passage, then nature without annoyance may well beare: and this is the cause why melancholicke persons are for the most part encumbred with costiuenesse, especially if they be leane withall, (as hardly are they otherwise) and want that natural basting of fat (which some haue more then sufficient) then is this hardnesse of stoole much more increased. The nourishment thus deliuered of this excrement, in the liuer is turned into bloud, & of white by farther processe of heat is made red. In passing of this triall it yeldeth two excrements, the one cholericke, and the other melancholicke, while it remaineth in the liuer, and before it be yet passed into the vaines; the cholericke is in her quantitie, except the meates and drinkes of them selues do minister greater store of that matter,

matter, else their bodies are vnapt for generatiõ of that humour; the melancholie is in great aboundance, by reason of the inclination of the complexion thereunto, & want of pure refining in the liuer; the aboundance wherof is such, that it passeth downe from the splene with grosse and melancholic iuyce into the Hemerodes, and deliuereth of pleurisies, phrensies, and madnesse, (wherto the melancholickes are subiect) if their flowe be not too sparing. This aboundance, and thicknesse causeth their splene to swell, which is sayd therefore to procure laughter, because it draweth, and sucketh the melancholicke excrement, and purgeth that humour which hath ben before declared to breed so many fearful passiõs and breedeth stoppings, whereby it defileth the whole supply of the humors. The bloud now discharged of the liuer, & possessed of the vains, yet leaueth another excremēt more liquid & thinne then the rest: this nature disburdeneth it selfe of by the vertue of the reins, whose office is to suck out that thinne humour, & to distill it into the bladder, frõ whence after a while nature remēbred therof, either by quantity, heat, or sharpnes deliuereth it quite out of the body. This excrement is not plentifull in melancholicke persons, but of colour white, by reason of colde, and litle stained for want of choler, & thicke of substance according to the bloud, frõ whence it is drawne. The bloud thus purified, and deliuered of so manie superfluous exerements, in the ende passeth from the great, into the small vaines, and from the small into the priuate poores of euery mem-

M iij

ber, and by diuerse degrees at the length receaueth the similitude of our nature, by the complexion of euerie part, and is vnited in all respectes vnto our natural substance. In this degree of natures worke, sundrie superfluities arise, partly common to all partes, aud partly priuate to certaine. The common is sweat, wherof melancholicke persons are spare, through drinesse, and sweat requiring heate working vpon a moisture, which both faile in the melancholicks. For want of sufficient heate they are not much annoyed that way, neither doth the humours of their bodies grosse of substance deliuer ready matter therunto. The other vniuersall kind is a kinde of insensible steme, which breatheth cōtinually frō our bodies, & appeareth on a mans shirt, though he haue not sweat & soiled it. This melancholick men haue more foule, then the other estates of bodie, and deliuer more plentie, especiallie if their bodies be chafed with exercise: for not hauing free passage otherwise, for causes before mentioned, it setleth about the skinne more aboundantly, and vppon exercise which openeth the poores, & rarifieth the bodie, maketh plaine an outward shewe. The particular excrements, especially worth noting, are that voyde from our head, stomach, and chest. From the head, melancholicke men haue abundance, by reason of the stomaches cruditie, whose vapors it congeleth, or gathereth into rhewme, and distilleth it into the mouth. From the stomach, it riseth by the graine of the throte, as you see moisture rise from the water pot by a clout in watering of millions,

lions & cucumbers. The longes voide not much although through want of heate it gathereth of crude excremēt in those parts, thicker, with lesse sense of heat, then moderate. These be the accidents which fall vnto melancholicke persons, & thus procured: if any haue bene omitted, either they be such as are of no moment to be knowne, or the reason of them is easily rendred frō that which hath of the rest bene shewne, neither was my purpose in precise manner to deliuer these points vnto you, as they are to be taught in a schoole of Philosophy, but only to giue you a tast of thē for better vnderstanding of your present state, and discharge of that duetie of friendship which your request layeth vpon me in this melancholicke theme. This far I haue proceeded in my discourse philosophically, in laying the whole case of melancholie (so far as my skill in nature extēdeth) before you, as the first part of your desire pretended: hereafter as the order of your request prescribeth, you shal haue mine opinion of that affection which riseth vpon horror, and conscience of sinne, with feare & feeling of Gods reuenging hand against the same; whether it be any part of melancholy or not; whether melancholick persons are subiect most therunto; what aduantage Satan taketh in this case by the frailtie of the bodie; with such other doubts, as your letter ministred vnto me; & in the end my counsell and comfort, and what direction else my physicke help wil afford, for restoring you to the former estate of your body, fallen in decay through this humour, and to that tranquillitie of minde, and those comfortes of Gods grace, which before this temptation assayled you, you ioyed in, and was able to minister comfort vnto others afflicted with like distresse; and so commit the successe of this my labour to the blessing of God, and referre my louing indeuour to that friendly acceptatiō, wherwith you are wont to value the slender offices of great good will vnto you.

Chap. XXXII.
Of the affliction of conscience for sinne.

OF all kinds of miseries that befall vnto man, none is so miserable as that which riseth of the sense of Gods wrath, and reuenging hand against the guiltie soule of a sinner. Other calamities afflict the body, and one part only of our nature: this the soule, which carieth the whole into societie of the same miserie. Such as are of the bodie, although they approch nigher the quicke then pouertie, or want of necessaries for maintenāce of this life, yet they faile in degree of misery, & come short of that which this forceth vpō the soule. The other touch those parts where the soule commandeth; pouertie, nakednesse, sicknesse and other of that kinde are mitigated with a minde resolute in patience, or indued with wisedome to ease that grieueth by supply of remedie: this sezeth vpon the seate of wisedome it selfe, and chargeth vpon all the excellencie of vnderstanding, and grindeth into powder all that standeth firme, and melteth like the dew before the Sunne whatsoeuer we reckē

of

OF MELANCHOLIE.

of a support of our defectes, and subdueth that wherwith all thinges else are of vs subdued: the cause, the guilt, the punishment, the reuenge, the ministers of the wrath, all concurring together in more forcible sort (& that against the vniuersall state of our nature, not for a time, but for euer) then in any other kind of calamitie whatsoeuer. Here the cause is not either woūd or surfet, shipwracke or spoile, infamie, or disgrace, but all kinde of misery ioyned together with a troubled spirit, feeling the beginnings, & expecting with desperat feare the eternall consummatiō of the indignatiō, & fierce wrath of Gods vengeāce against the violation of his holy cōmandemēts: which although in this life it taketh not away the vse of outward benefits, yet doth the internal anguish bereue vs of all delight of thē, & that pleasant relish they are indued with to our comforts: so that manifold, better were it the vse of thē were quite takē away, thē for vs in such sort to enioy them. Neither is here the guiltines of breach of humane lawes (whose punishment extendeth no farther then this present life, which euen of it selfis full of calamities not much inferiour to the paine adioyned vnto the transgression of ciuill lawes) but of the Law diuine, & the censure executed with the hand of God, whose fierce wrath prosecuteth the punishment eternally as his displeasure is like to him selfe, and followeth vs into our graues, & receaueth no satisfaction with anie punishment, either in regard of continuance or of extremitie. Such is the crime, and such is the guiltinesse which infer the reward fitting and fully answering the desert: which being a seaparation from Gods fauour the creator and blesser of all thinges, the fountaine of all peace and comforte, what creature the worke of his handes dare cheere vs with any consolation? or what assurance may we haue of escape if we would flee? the punishment as it hath no misery to compare with, and the sence thereof not to be described to the capacity of any, but of such as haue felt the anguish, as your selfe at this present, is rather to be shewed by negation of all happines, then by direct affirmation of torment. For as the happines rising of Gods fauour, besides the enioying of all bodely and earthly blessinges, so farre forth as is expedient for vs, and tending to his glory, is aboue al conceite of mans heart, and reporte of tunge: so the contrary estate exceedeth all vnderstanding of the minde, and vtteraunce of speach, and is such as it is aboue measure vnhappy and most miserable, inflicted by Gods reuenge, who is himself a consuming fire, and whose wrath once kindled, burneth to the bottome of hell. In other miseries of execution, the minister may vpon cōpassion and entreaty mitigate the rigor: here Sathan moued with the old ranchor, and an ennimy vnrecōcilable hath the charge, who is so far of from pitying our estate, that to the encrease of torment, where the Lord chasteneth with mercy, and limiteth sometimes this tormentor in compasse of our possessions and goods, he vrgeth skinne for skinne, streatch out thy hand, touch his bones and his flesh: and if expresse

charge

charge were not to the contrary would not satisfie himselfe therewith, except life, yea not only temporall, but that euerlasting, whereof we haue assured promises of God, wet also for payment. But what doe I describe this vnto you, whose present experience exceedeth my discourse? Although it be necessary to be laid open, for more cleare distinguishing thereof from the melancholy passions aboue mentioned, and the quality of this miserie thus being knowne, such as by Godds mercy are yet free, may acknowledge his grace therein, pray for the continewance of that freedome, and pittie the estate of such as grone vnder the burthen of that heauy crosse, wherein no reason is able to minister cōsolatiō, nor the burthen wherof the Angels thēselues haue ability to sustaine. Leauing the description of this affliction I will fall to the deliberation, whether this kinde be of melancholie or not, and so proceede to the doubtes, which the comparison of them both together may minister vnto vs.

Chap. XXXIII.
VVhether the conscience of sinne and the affliction thereof be melancholy or not.

BY that hath bene before declared it may easily appeare the affliction of soule through cōscience of sinne is quite another thing then melācholy: but yet to the end it may lie most cleare, I will lay them together, so shall their distinct natures thus compared bewray the error of some,

and the prophanes of otherſome, who either accompt the cauſe naturall, melancholy, or madnes, or elſe hauing ſome farther inſighte, with a
Stoicall prophanes of Atheiſme, skoffe at that
kinde of afflictiō, againſt which they themſelues
labour to ſhut vp their hard heartes, & with ob-
ſtinacie of ſtomack to beare out that whereof
they tremble with horror, and not hauing other
refuge, paſſe ouer the ſenſe with a deſperat reſo-
lution: which would awake, and doth not faile at
times, to touch the quick of the ſecureſt, & moſt
flinty harted gallantes of the world. Therfore to
the end, the one may be reformed in their iudg-
ment, and the other may thereby take occaſion
to reforme their maners, let them conſider that
this is a ſorrow and feare vpon cauſe, & that the
greateſt cauſe that worketh miſery vnto mā: the
other contrarily a meere fancy & hath no groūd
of true and iuſt obiect, but is only raiſed vpō diſ-
order of humour in the fancy, and raſhly deliuered to the heart, which vpon naturall credulity
faireth in paſſion, as if that were in deede wherof the fancy giueth a falſe larume. In this the body ſtandeth oft times in firme ſtate of health,
perfect in complexion, and perfect in ſhape, & al
ſymmetrie of his partes, the humors in quantitie
and quality not exceeding nor wanting their naturall proportion. In the other, the complexiō is
depraued, obſtructions hinder the free courſe of
ſpirits & humors, the blood is ouer groſſe, thick,
& impure, & nature ſo diſordered, that diuerſe
melancholicke perſons haue iudged themſelues
ſome earthie pitchers, otherſome cockes, other
ſome

some to haue wanted their heades &c, as if they had bin transported by the euill quality of the humor into straunge natures: here the sēses are oft times perfect both outward & inward, the imagination sound, the heart well compact & resolute, & this excepted, want no courage. In the other, the inward sense and outward to feebled, the fancy ouertaken with gastly fumes of melācholy, and the whole force of the spirite closed vp in the dungion of melancholy darkenes, imagineth all darke, blacke and full of feare, their heartes are either ouertender and rare, & so easily admitte the passion, or ouer closse of nature serue more easily to imprison, the chearefull spirites the causes of comforte to the rest of the bodie: whereby they are not in one respect only fainte harted, and full of discourage: but euerie smal occasion, yea though none be, they are driuen with tide of that humour to feare, euē in the middest of security. Here it first proceedeth frō the mindes apprehension: there from the humour, which deluding the organicall actions, abuseth the minde, and draweth it into errionious iudgement, through false testimony of the outward reporte. Here no medicine, no purgation, no cordiall, no tryacle or balme are able to assure the afflicted soule and trembling heart, now painting vnder the terrors of God: there in melancholy the vayne opened, neesing powder or bearefoote ministred, cordialls of pearle, Saphires, and rubies, with such like, recomforte the heart throwne downe, & appaled with fatasticall feare. In this affliction, the perill is not of body, and corporall actions, or decay of seruile, and temporall vses, but of the whole nature soule and body cut of from the life of God, and from the sweet influence of his fauour, the fountaine of all happines and eternall felicity. Finally if they be diligētly cōpared in cause, in effect, in quality, in whatsoeuer respect these vnreuerent and prophane persons list to match them, they shall appeare of diuerse nature, neuer to be be coupled in one felowship, as more particularly shalbe shewed hereafter. The cause here is the seuerity of Gods iudgement, summoning the guilty consciēce: the subiect is the sinnefull soule apprehending the terror thereof, which is not momentary or for a season, but for euer and euer: the issue of this affliction is eternall punishment, satisfactory to the iustice of the eternall God, which is endlesse, and whose seuerity admitteth no mediation, neither that extended to one ioynte, sinue or vaine, but to all, neither that of the body only, but of the soule, whose nature, as it is impatible of all other thinges, and of all other thinges in greatest peace, assurance and tranquillitye, so once shaken by the terrours of Gods wrath, and blasted with that whirlewinde of his displeasure, falleth and with it driueth the whole frame of our nature into extreame miserie and vtter confusion: so farre they are abused who iudge these cases as naturall, and such is the calamity of those whom the prophane ones of this world propound vnto themselues as matter of scoffe and derision, laboring by al meanes to benumme the sense of that stinge, which sinne

euer

Of Melancholie.

euer carrieth in the tayle, what pretence so euer it sheweth of right, profit or pleasure, in face of outward appearance, to delude the foole & simple in his wayes, skillfull to do euill, sottish in the pathes of righteousnes, and vtterly ignorant of her rule, and wherein nature giueth some sparke of light, more distinctly to discerne, euen there with corruption of affection, like to stubburne & vnbroaken horse, shaketh of reason, dispiseth her manage, and layeth the noble ryder in the dust. In respect of you my deare *M*. I know this discourse were superfluous, who standeth in neede of salue to the sore, and beareth not the least touch of this gale, but because my purpose in this labour is not only to informe and to comforte you, but also for the instruction of others, beare with this, and passe it ouer, as not belonging vnto you, but to the foole: of whome Solomon speaketh, that followeth wickednes like an Oxe that goeth to the slaughter, and as a foole to the stockes for correction, and as a bird hasteth to the snare, not knowing that he is in daūger. Touching your particular estate, that you may iudge thereof more sincerely, you are to esteeme of it, as mixed of the melancholick humour and that terror of God: which as it is vpon thē wicked an entrance into their eternall destructiō, so vnto you, it is, (as I shall hereafter at large make proofe) a fatherly frowning only for a time, to correct that which in you is to be reformed, and an admonition of farther circumspection in your wayes and course of life hereafter. For the first pointe you may remember your swolne splene, with windnes and hardenes vnder the left ribbes, the hemeroydes not flowing according to their vsuall manner, the blacknes and grossenes of that blood which hath ben taken from you vpon occasion, your dreames ordinarily fearefull, your solitarines and exceeding sadnes, with almost all kinde of accidentes which accompanie melancholy. For the other part whereof most you complaine, the manner leadeth me to iudge thereof otherwise then naturall, both because such is indeede the feare & terror of God sent vpon man, and no effect of any creature or cause besides: as also because the obiect or mouing cause is, in reason and cleare vnderstanding, voide of all abuse of fancy, such as of necessity inforceth these lamentable effects which your soule feeleth & desireth the release of, vpon you the crosse falleth more heauily, in so much as you are vnder the disaduantage of the melancholicke complexion: whose opportunity Sathan embraceth to vrge all terror against you to the fall. But remember that he who hath redeemed vs, passed vnder these feares & hath sanctified them to his redeemed, and according to his example, who was heard in that which he feared, when in the dayes of his flesh he did offer vp prayers and supplications with strög crying and teares vnto him that was able to saue him from death: so follow him in hope and patience, who hath obtained the victory not for him selfe onely, but for all such as in like temptation depend vpon him. To the end my labour may giue you a more perfect direction in this heauy case,

case, what is naturall, and what is according to the good pleasure of God in the other distresse aboue nature, I will make particular distinction of both in the Chapter following, to your clearer vnderstanding.

Chap. XXXIIII.
The particular difference betwixt melancholy, & the distressed conscience in the same person.

WHatsoeuer molestation riseth directly as a proper obiect of the mind, that in that respect is not melancholicke, but hath a farther ground then fancie, and riseth from conscience, condemning the guiltie soule of those ingrauen lawes of nature, which no man is voide of, be he neuer so laborous. This is it, that hath caused the prophane poëts to haue fained Hecates Eumenides, and the infernall furies; which although they be but fained persons, yet the matter which is shewed vnder their maske, is serious, true, and of wofull experience. This taketh nothing of the body, nor intermedleth with humour, but giueth a direct wounde with those firie dartes, which men so afflicted make their mone of. Of this kinde Saule was possessed, to whom the Lord sent an euill spirite to encrease the torment; and Iudas the traytor, who tooke the reuenge of betraying the innocent vppon him selfe with his owne handes; such was the anguish that Esau felte when he found no repentance, after he had sold his birthright for a messe of pottage; and such is the estate of all defiled consciences with hainous crimes; whose harts are neuer free from that worme, but with deadly bite thereof are driuen to dispaire. These terrible obiectes which properly appertaine vnto the minde, are such as onely affect it with horror of Gods iustice for breach of those lawes naturall, or written in his word, which by duty of creation, we are holden to obey. For the minde as it is impatible of anie thing but of God onely that made it, so standeth it in awe of none but of him, neither admitteth it any other violence then from him, into whose handes it is most terrible and fearefull to fall. This causeth such distresse vnto those that feele the torment hereof, that they would redeeme it gladly, if it were possible with anie other kind, yea mith suffering all other kind of miserie. This hath befallen vnto the wisest among men while the integritie of their vnderstanding hath stood sound; it taketh of a sodaine like lightning, and giueth no warning. Here the puritie of the bloud, and the sinceritie and liuelinesse of the spirits auayle nothing to mitigate the paine, but onely the expiatorie sacrifice of the vnspotted lambe. On the contrarie part, when anie conceit troubleth you that hath no sufficient grounde of reason, but riseth onely vpon the frame of your brayne, which is subiect (as hath bene before shewed) vnto the humour, that is right melancholicke, & so to be accopted of you. These are false points of reason deceaued by the melancholie braine, and disguised scarres of the heart, without abilitie to worke the pretenced annoyaunce: neither

ther do they approch the substaunce, and the substantiall and soueraigne actions of the soule, as the other doeth. This estate happeneth by degrees, and getteth strength in time, to the encumbrance of all the instrumentall actions, and driue the braine into a sottishnesse, and obscure the cleare light of reason. Here the humour purged, and the spirite attenuate and refreshed with remedie conuenient, the brayne strengthened, and the hart comforted with cordialls, are meanes most excellent ordayned of God for this infirmitie. And to deliuer you in a word the difference, whatsoeuer is besides conscience of sinne in this case, it is melancholie: which conscience terrified, is of such nature, so beset with infinite feares and distrust, that it easilie wasteth the pure spirit, congeleth the liuely bloud, and striketh our nature in such sort, that it soone becommeth melancholicke, vile and base, and turneth reason into foolishnesse, and disgraceth the beautie of the countenance, and transformeth the stoutest Nabucadnezar in the world into a brute beast; so easily is the body subiect to alteration of minde, & soone looseth with anguish and distruction thereof, all the support of his excellencie. Besides this in you, vaine feares, and false conceits of apparitions, imagination of a voyce sounding in your eares, frightfull dreames, distrust of the consumption, and putrifying of one part or other of your bodie, & the rest of this crue, are causes of molestation, which are whelpes of that melancholicke litter, & are bred of the corrupted state of the body al-

altered in spirit, in bloud, in substance and complexion, by the aboundance of this settling of the bloud, which we call melancholie. This increaseth the terrour of the afflicted minde, doubling the feare & discouragement,& shutteth vp the meanes of consolatiō, which is after another sort to be conueyed to the minde, then the way which the temptation taketh to breed distrust of Gods mercy,& pardon. For that hath sinne the meanes, which needeth no conueyaunce, but is bred with vs,& entreth euen into our conceptiō: neither is the guiltinesse brought vnto vs by foreine report, but the knowledge riseth from the conscience of the offender: the meanes (I meane the outwarde meanes of consolation and cure) must needs passe by our senses to enter the mind whose instrument being altred by the humor, & their sincerity stained with the obscure and dark spots of melancholy, receiue not indifferētly the medicine of cōsolatiō. So it both mistaketh, that which it apprehendeth, and deliuereth it imperfectly to the minds consideratiō. As their brains are thus euill disposed, so their harts in no better case,& acquainted with terror,& ouerthrown with that fearful passiō, hardly set free the cherfull spirits, feebled with the corporall prison of the body, & hardly yeeld to persuasion of comfort what soeuer it bringeth of assurance. This causeth the release of the affliction to be long & hard, and not answerable to the swiftnesse of the procuring cause, hauing so many wayes top asse, & encountring so many lets before it meet with the sore. For as the cause respecteth not time nor

place,

place, no circumstance of perſon, nor condition, ſeeketh no opportunity of corporall imbecillity, but breakeath through all ſuch conſiderations, & beareth downe all reſiſtance: ſo the comfort requireth them all agreable, & miſſing any one, worketh feble effects,& ſlow. Here the coforters perſon, his maner, the time, & place, may hinder the conſolatiõ: here the braine & hart, being as it were the gates & entraunce vnto the ſoule, as they be affected, ayd, or hinder the conſolatiõ;ſo that the conſciēce diſtreſſed falling into a melācholy ſtate of body, therby receiueth delay of reſtoring in reſpect of outward meanes; though the grace of God, & his mercy, his comfortable ſpirit, & gracious fauor in like ſwiftneſſe without meanes may reſtore the minde thus diſtreſſed: which lieth equally open to the kind of cure, euē as it lay to the wound. Thus I coclude this point of difference, & marke betwixt melancholy and the ſoules proper anguiſh, whoſe only cauſe proceedeth from Gods vengeance & wrath apprehended of the guilty ſoule: neither doth melancholy alone, (though it may hinder the outward meanes of conſolation, as it hath bin before ſhewed) any thing make men more ſubiect vnto this kind of afflictiõ. Firſt becauſe the body worketh nothing vpon the ſoule altogether impatible of any other ſauing of God alone. 2. The torment is ſuch as riſeth frõ an efficient that requireth no diſpoſitiõ of means; God himſelf. 3. The cõſort is not procured by any corporal inſtrumēts, ſo neither is the diſcõfort procured or increaſed that way; moreouer the cauſe, the ſubiect, the proper effects are other then corporall. For although in that case the hart is heauy, deliuering a passió answerable to the fearfull apprehension, yet the sense of those that are vnder this crosse feele an anguish farre beyond all afflictió of naturall passion coupled with that organicall feare and heauinesse of heart. The melancholy disposeth to feare, doubt, distrust, & heauinesse, but all either without cause, or where there is cause aboue it inforceth the passion. Here both the most vehement cause vrgeth, and alwayes carieth a passió therwith aboue the harts affection, euen the entry of those torments, which cánot be cóceaued at full, as our nature now stádeth, nor deliuered by report. Here in this passion, the cause is not feare nor passionate griefe, but a torment procuring these affections: and euen as the punishment of bodily racking is not the passion of the hart, but causeth it only; so the hart fareth vnder this sore of the mind, which here properlie fretteth and straineth the sinnes of the soule, wherefrom the heart taketh his grieuous discouragement, and fainteth vnder Gods iustice. Hitherto you haue described that which your soule feeleth, not to instruct you, but that other may more truly iudge of the case, and the distinction betwixt melancholy & it, may be more apparant.

Chap. xxxv.
The affliction of mind to what persons it befalleth, and by what meanes.

Although no man is by nature freed fró this affliction, in so much as all men are sinners,
and

and being culpable of the breach of God lawes, incurre the punishment of condemnation: yet is the melancholicke person more then any subiect therunto: not that the humor hath such power, which hath before bin declared to stand far a loofe of such effect, but by reason the melacholicke person is most doubtfull, & iclous of his estate, not only of this life, but also of the life to come; this maketh him fall into debate with him selfe, & to be more then curious; who finding his actions not fitting the naturall, or written line of righteousnesse, & wāting that archpiller of faith & assurance in Christ Iesus our hope, partly thorough feare findeth the horror, and partly (if it please God so far to touch) feeleth the verie anguish due vnto the sinner, & in that most miserable condition falleth into flat dispaire. This commeth to passe, when the curious melancholy carieth the minde into the senses of such misteries as exceed humayne capacity, and is desirous to know more thē is reuealed in the word of truth: or being ignorant of that which is reuealed thorough importunate inquirie, of a sudden falleth into that gulfe of Gods secret counselles which swalloweth vp all conceit of man or angell: and measuring the trueth of such depth of misteries by the shallow modill of his owne wit, is caught & deuoured of that which his presumptuous curiositie moued him to attempt to apprehend. Of melancholy persons, especially such as are most contemplatiue, except they be well grounded in the word of God, & remoue not one haire therfrom in their speculations, are this wayes most

ouertaken, & receaue the punishment of ouer-bold attēpt of those holy things, which the Lord hath reserued to his owne counsell: while they neglect the declared truth, propounded for rule of life and practise, in written wordes reuealed; not remembring the exhortation of Moyses to the children of Israell: the secrets are the Lords but the reuealed will, apperteineth to vs, & our children. And this in mine opinion is one cause wherefore melancholicke personnes are more prone to fall into this pitte, then such as are in their organicall members otherwise affected. Nowe contemplations are more familiar with melancholicke persons then with other, by reason they be not so apt for action, consisting also of a temper still and slowe according to the nature of the melancholie humour, which if it be attenuated with heate, deliuereth a drie, subtile and pearcing spirite, more constant and stable then anie other humour, which is a great helpe to this contemplation. As the melancholicke is most subiect to the calamitie before mentioned, and especially the contemplatine, so of them most of all, such whose vocation consisteth in studie of hard pointes of learning, and that philosophicall (especially of Nature) haue cause in this case to carie a lowe saile, and sometime to strike, and lay at the anker of the Scriptures of God, lest by tempest of their presumption, they be caried into that whirle poole, whereout they be in daunger (without the especiall grace of Gods mercie) neuer to deliuer them selues. Such except they be well ballaced with knowledge

OF MELANCHOLIE.

ledge of the Scriptures, and assurance of Gods spirite, are neuer able to abide the oughtnesse of their sinnes, when they shall be once vnfolden, and the narrowe point of reprobation and election propounded vnto their melancholicke braines and hearts, and most miserale polluted soules: vnacquainted with Gods couenaunt of mercie, and that earnest of his fauour, the comfortable spirit of his grace. Of such as haue some knowledge in the worde, and practise of obedience, the want of the true apprehending of gods reuealed wil touching election and reprobation, and the right method of learning & conceauing the doctrine, causeth some to stumble, and fall at this stone. For as a sworde taken at the wrong end is readie to wound the hand of the taker, & held by the handle is a fit weapon of defence; euen so the doctrine of predestination being preposterously conceiued, may through fault of the conceiuer procure hurt; whereas of it selfe it is the most strong rocke of assurance, in all stormes of temptations that can befall vnto bodie or soule. The one part of predestination, is Gods immutable will, the cause and rule of all iustice, and vttermost of all reason in his workes: the other part is the execution of that will, according to mercie or iustice, sauing or condemning, with all the meanes thereto belonging: Christ. Iesus in those of whom the Lorde will shewe mercie, and the iust desert of a sinner on whome he is determined to shewe the iustice of his wrath. If this most comfortable doctrine, and the same ancher of our profession be not in all partes equally apprehended, we may not onely misse the benefite therof through our owne fault, but receiue wounde and daungerous hurte thereby. For if the consideration be bent vpon Gods will and counsel only, without respect of the means, it is impossible but the frailty of mans nature must needes be distracted into diuerse perilous and desperate feares, finding nothing in it selfe that may answere his iustice, and withstand the fearefull sentence of condemnation: if it stay in the meanes of his iustice only, and haue not eye vpon his mercy in his sonne Christ, then likewise ariseth an assurance of eternall destruction to the consciēce defiled, and the guilty soule deformed with iniquity: if the meanes of his mercy be regarded without farther respect of his eternall decree and immouable iustice, then is there also no assurance of his mercy vnto miserable man, who melteth like snow and vanisheth like a vapour before his iustice, and doubting of the continuance of his fauour alwayes hangeth in suspence. All these considerations thus seuerally falling into the melancholick person, moue doubt and care, and either breed a resolute desperatnes, or a continuall distrust, tossing hither and thither the soule not established by knowledge and faith in Gods eternall counsell, & the most wise, iust and mercifull meanes of his execution: which being perfectly knowne according to the word, and sealed vp in the christian heart by the worke of Gods spirite, is so farre of from disquieting the spirit or breeding doubt, that the children of God in all temptations finde the immutability

OF MELANCHOLIE.

mutability of Gods counsell, and the testimony of his fauour in their consciences by his spirite, to supporte them in all stormes of temptation, and to be the rocke against which no violence of Sathan, or his ministers, or whatsoeuer their owne infirmity offereth of discouragement can preuaile. Besides these, such as read the word of God with passionate humour, fall into this inconuenience: especially if without guide and instruction they carie any presumption of minde and are not modest and warie in their collections, such being melancholicke may easily fall into distrust of Gods mercy, & perish in dispaire. So that ignorance and infidelity, are the chiefe causes of this miserable estate: whereinto many haue fallen, especially such as haue neuer bene able to be recomforted, which for the most part are they who with neglect of Godds feare and hardnes of heart, against their conscience and knowledge, haue with desperate purpose gathered strength in the wayes of sinne, and haue cast of all remorse, til the Lordes vengeaunce in this sort ouertake them, or haue fallen into that sinn whereof the Apostle speaketh of, that none should pray for, and which our Sauiour calleth the sinne against the holy Ghost. Other some ther be (of which number I know you deare *M*.) that fearing the Lord with sincerity of hearte, haue bene notwithstanding this way distressed, the weight of their sinnes exceeding for a time the strength of their faith, whose case I take to be thus farre, other then such as I haue before mentioned: euen as in stormie tempest the ship stirreth at euery blast and sourge of the sea to be in daunger of wrack, and the yong ash bending to euery blast of winde, seemeth in perill of breaking & rooting vp, whē both the ship kepeth her constant course, & the tree yet hath his rooting; so in you, & those of your disposition in this case, the tempest, and storme of this temptation, raysed partly by your owne weakenes, and partely through Sathans tempestious malice: causeth your faith to bend, and seeme feeble, & yeelding to this force, while notwithstanding you be built on the rocke, & planted with the hand of God in the Eden of his gracious election, & remayne a plante for euer in his paradise of eternall felicitie. Such (as you your self) herin offend, that you measure your selues by your infirmities, which hath so farre vse in vs to breed a watchfull care ouer our owne wayes, & not to discourage vs: & consider that we are as the Lord esteemeth, who is more glorified in shewing mercie, thē in executing of his wrath: whose word declareth vnto vs, that he loued vs being ennemies, and found vs whē we were lost, and loathed not our polution, but for himselfe onely offered his mercy: so that we must stand in that reckning of our selues which the Lord will haue vs to doe in his mercie: else shal we be wrōg iudges of the wayes of the Almighty. Euen as one that hath not had experience of trauaile by sea, feareth euery weauing of the ship, & doubteth of perill, where the nature of the trauailer is such without hazard or daunger; So you, & such as are in like case afflicted, imagine euery puffe of this kinde of tēptation

OF MELANCHOLIE.

eation to be nothing else but the gate of destruction, when as notwithstanding it is the verie course & way where through God doth lead his dearest children: whose counsells are not to be measured, by our infirmities, nor by that we cast, forecast, or doubt, but as he himselfe hath pronoūced of his own wayes, & as many of his children haue proued before vs. Here the melācholie taketh aduantage and Sathan prosecuteth a maine, w̄ bēding your affectiōs to feare, doubt, & distrust, stoppeth that consolation the mercy of god affordeth, & which his childrē are ready to minister vnto you. And these are melancholickes of another sort; who notwithstanding they endeuour to feare God, yet not aduised, through this base & vile humor, receiue discouragemēt in thēselues more then (through Gods mercie) they haue need, til such time as the cōfort of his spirite by due means, & alteration of their body by cōueniēt remedy of the godly phisician raise thē vp againe. These are melācholiks most disposed, by reason of the euill temper of their bodies to this affliction, not by power of the humor, which resteth in their bodies, & toucheth not the minde, but by reasō they are more curious & distrustfull thē other cōplexiōs: which being ioyned with ignorance, or a preposterous knowledge cast thē into these laberinthes of spirituall sorow, whereout very hardly are they at the length able to dispatch themselues without great mercy of God, and diligent and carefull applying of his meanes. But you may say vnto me, can a man by his owne power drawe on this kinde of crosse, which you haue before declared to be the hand of God? yea verily, if Gods only mercie be not his stay, euen as our first parents voluntarily gaue their neckes, and in them all their posterity vnder the yoke of Sathan: and as the vengeance of Gods iustice alwayes burneth against the wicked, & his sword continually employed, which nothing cā quéch but the water of his grace flowing from the sids of his Sonne, and that spiritual complet armour whereof S. Paul speaketh of: so should euen all of vs in this life taste of the heate, & feele the dint of that sword, if his mercy in his Sonne & for his Saintes cause on the earth, he staied not the ielousie of his wrath: His anger our sinnes pull on, but his mercy is only for himselfe. Thus you haue heard what manner affliction this of the minde and conscience of sinne, not comforted by assurance of pardon is, how it differeth from melancholy, how melancholicke persons are most subiect therunto, and by what meanes this calamity is procured, with the diuersity of persons thus afflicted: hereafter you shall vnderstand (which is your chiefe desire) my counsell and cure, both in that state of minde wherin you stand, and whereof the Lord graunt you speedy and comfortable release, and also in what your crased body surgayned with melancholy and all his vncomfortable accidentes doth of naturall & phisick help of medicine require. But first my deare M. giue way to my wordes of comfort, and for the old friendships sake, and sweete society we haue had in times past, alwayes seasoned

with

with heauenly meditations and spirituall conferences, denie me not that intereſt which ſhalbe both comfortable vnto you, and ioyfull to many of your friendes, whoſe prayers are with ſobbes powred out for your releaſe: eſpecially beware leaſt vnaduiſedly you diſhonour god in this kind of ſorow, who is the God of peace and comfort.

Chap. xxx.
A conſolation vnto the afflicted conſcience.

YOu feele (you ſay) the wrath of God kindled againſt your ſoule, and anguiſh of conſcience moſt intollerable, and can finde (notwithſtanding continuall prayers and inceſſaunt ſupplication made vnto the Lord) no releaſe, & in your owne iudgement ſtand reprobate from Gods couenant, and voide of all hope of his inheritance, expecting the conſummation of your miſery and fearefull ſentence of eternall condēnation: I pray you (deare brother) conſider Gods mercies of old, and the former experience of his fauour, and thoſe holy teſtimonies of election which you haue in times paſt made plentifully ſhew of, and conſider whether it be not rather a temptation, then as you imagine, Gods anger againſt you. Of temptations there are diuerſe ſortes, ſome riſing frō our owne natures, otherſome from without vs: ſuch as are without our natures, either ſpringe from our malitious enemie Sathan, or from ſuch allurementes, or terrors which the world toſſeth vs withall: In theſe

Sathan is a worker, besides his owne peculiar manner of tempting. His temptations are either by corporall possession, or with more liberty and freedome to the tempted. Of our owne natures springe the temptations which rise of the roote of originall sinne, without any forraine instigation from the world, whatsoeuer is either a bayte of pleasure, or fright of terror, which increase the actuall sinnes springing from the originall roote, and lay as it were compasse, and powreth on water, to that vngracious stock. Now if this your affliction be no other, but some kinde of these téptatiõs (which I haue no doubt to make manifest and playne vnto you) then are you to esteeme of your case more comfortably thẽ you do, and to attend with patience the issue, which not onely is not infallible to signifi: determinatly of election or reprobation, but in such as are of like conuersation vnto you, and haue giuen euident testimonies of a sound faith groũded vpõ knowledge, as you haue done, bringeth forth the fruites of patience, experience, hope, increase of faith, and not onely in the end yeeldeth plenty of spirituall ioy, and comforte vnto themselues, but furnisheth also with power, and hability to confirme others, both by their owne example, and wordes of great consolation from their owne experience. In all the former kindes of temptations, there is hope, and examples are sundry in ech kinde: of which the corporall inhabiting of Sathan is the greatest, fullest of tertour and dispaire: yet the history of the deedes and sayinges of Christ, the wrytinges of the E-

uangelist

uangelifts do teftifie of whole legions difpoffeſſed of that habitation, by the power of Chrift mercifully extended vpon such poore and miserable captiues; which examples are written for our inſtruction againſt like times of affliction, that we giue not ouer hope, though millions of deuills ſhould poſſeſſe vs within, and enuirone vs without; but knowe his power is aboue all force of the enemie, and his mercie farre ſurmounting Sathans malice. But before I proceede in this particular, I will make plaine demonſtration vnto you, that you haue no cauſe in this ſorte to feare, nor haue anie ſhadowe of grounde whereon you ſhould reſolue againſt your ſelfe vppon the poynt of reprobation, but that theſe moleſtations and terrours, which you nowe indure are temptations, rather for your farther good and profite, then grounded reſolutions, of ſuch lamentable iſſue : which hauing declared vnto you in the generalitie, I will enter into the particular kindes, wherewith I iudge you are thus diſtreſſed. Firſt I will endeuour to looſe the holde your melancholie hath layed vppon the aſſuraunce (as you take it) of reprobation; which hauing firſt perfourmed, your iudgement may more eaſilie embrace the other parte, which is a tryall onely for a time, and a meere temptation. Although Gods children euerie one haue their ſaluation founded vppon his eternall decree of mercie towardes them, publiſhed by the preaching of the Goſpell, and written, and ſealed in the heart of his choſen, by the power of the ſpirite of adop-

O

tion, which crieth Abba, father, and testifieth in measure, some more & some lesse, according to the dispensatiō of that grace; yet on the contrarie part, there is no euident and vndoubted signe of reprobation in any, while they liue: (because there may be hope of repentance) but onely that sinne, which Christ calleth the sinne against the holie Ghost, and for which the Apostle forbiddeth to pray: this the Diuines do expound to be an open & wilfull apostasie from God, with malitious hate against the profession of his knowen trueth. Next vnto this sinne, is impenitencie: which can not be knowne, till death make shewe thereof, and cut of time of repentance. Of the first of these, examples are verie rare, as Iulianus the Emperour called apostata: of the other, Cain, Esau, Saul, Iudas, and the prophane people of the world that know not Christ, and such as knowe him onely in vaine profession outwardly, and so continue, are patternes of the sinne, and shall be examples of Gods vengeance. But first touching that sinne, wherefore no prayer is to be made, (because it witnesseth, and sealeth vp reprobation to the offender in this life) I will by comparinge your course of life, and your present demeanour with that sinne, manifestly lay open your case to be farre other then reprobate. Before I enter hereinto, you must beware you make no mo sinnes of that kind, then God him selfe hath pronounced to be of that sort: for in these matters that concerne Gods religion, euen the perfection of our wisedome is but follie, much more our sicke

braines,

braines, and melancholicke vnderstanding, is farre to be remoued from handling such holie thinges, whereof none can geue rule, but he who knoweth the perfect nature, (as I may so speake) of God, which is knowen onely to him selfe; so that here you must rest in this case, and striue to see with no sharper eye, then so farre as God hath reuealed; nor enter other course in search of such matters of his secresie, then he hath him selfe manifested: by whose Oracles we are instructed, that only one kinde of sinne cutteth of all hope of saluation in such as haue professed Christ, and that only becaufe it is of such nature, that it closeth vp all remorse of repentaunce: being the height of all iniquitie, equall with that of the deuilles them selues, who are shut out of Gods fauour for euer. If this then be the onely sinne which brandeth the wicked soule to eternall condemnation, and you (deare heart) haue not in anie sort thus offended, (as I haue no doubt to make euident proofe) whie do you vnkindlie torment your owne heart, and throwe your selfe into that pit of destruction, from which the Lord hath redeemed you? and as though you were your owne and not his, a possession of your own purchase to be bestowed as fancie leadeth you, and not Gods creation, wrought by his spirite of regeneration, ordayned for his seruice and glorie. Nowe let vs enter into the consideration, whether you haue sinned against the holie Ghost or not: which if you haue in deede done (as peraduenture your humour would leade you) where is the renouncing of Gods religion, which you haue hitherto professed and presently do hartely embrace? Where is that malice, which prosecuteth this mischiefe? What persecution haue you in word or deede raised against the truth? What sword haue you euer drawne against it, or what volumes haue you written against sound doctrine, with purposed opposition against your own conscience, neither that of frailtie, but of meere will and obstinacie? If your humour be not able to alleadge such testimonies, (as it cannot in deed, these thinges being matters of iudgement and will, and not of fancie, and consisting of euidencie to be knowen of others, and not of imaginacie conceit of a fearful and distrustfull hart) giue ouer I pray you these melancholicke priudices against your selfe, and prepare your heart to receaue comfort, which the word of promise ministreth vnto you. For that sinne except onely, all other are within compasse of grace, and haue no power to shut vs from Gods fauour. Be it that you haue sinned against your conscience; yet certaine, condemnation and casting of, doth not necessarily ensue thereupon; else should there be not a person on whome God should shewe mercie. For we all sinne in that manner, and the good we would (our conscience bearing witnesse of our duetie, and breach of that we are bounde to do) we do not; but the sinne which we would not do in respect of regeneration, that we commit through our frailtie, which groweth vp in strenghth, by increases of God to perfesection, and hath euermore in it not to discou-

rage

rage vs, but to breede circumspection, and to remember vs where our perfection and excellencie lieth, euen without vs, in that vnspotted lambe Christ Iesus. For our willes are corrupted, not onely in that they are seduced by corrupt iudgement, which is the least part of their want; but when contrarie to iudgement grounded either vppon nature, or the plaine worde of trueth, we make choyce of that we knowe is naught, or preferre the greater euill before the lesse. Otherwise should our nature obtaine in this life a greater perfection, then our first parentes had in paradice, whose freedome of will was peruerted to that, which was against the knowen commaundement of God: and giue any one facultie or practise of the minde be perfect, all must needs be of like purenesse; seeing equallie they were corrupted, and equallie receaue restauration. This perfection we are to hope for, and attende the consummation of the rudimentes of righteousnesse, which both in knowledge and vse are in part blind and impotent, and in heauen are to receaue the absolute perfection and beautie, fully agreeable to Gods good will and vprightnesse of his iustice. If then you haue neither sinned against the holie Ghost, which is plaine through manifold testimonies of vnfaigned faith, euen at this time being full of sighes and groanes for your offences, carefull to eschue what soeuer is repugnaunt to Gods will, releeuinge with tender affection of Christian loue the necessities of others; neither in the whole course of your life, hauing bene of notorious marke of iniquitie, much lesse a blasphemer of that holie name, and a renouncer, with contumelie of the holie profession: assure your selfe that your present estate is no other, but a storme of temptation, and no marke of perdition) from which the Lorde, (after triall of faith and patience) will deliuer you, and sende that calme peace and tranquillitie, which in times past you haue enioyed, and shall by his grace againe recouer, to your euerlasting comfort. Of temptations some touch our fayth, and other some the fruites thereof. Our faith; as whether we beleeue or not. The fruites: either of profession of the truth, when persecution or feare, or fauour of men, slaken our zeale, and smother the outwarde shewe of those glorious graces of faith, & of the spirite, or in the fruites of obedience sutable and kindly vnto our profession, as those which concerne persons, possessions, or name, wherein charitie towarde men is broken: all these temptations, though both affection do incline vnto them, (excepting incredulitie, which bringeth foorth impenitencie, and renunciation of the faith) and will bring them to effect, yet are they not of power to separate vs from the loue of God in Christ, whose sacrifice is all sufficient, and propitiatorie for all kindes of sinne, (that onely before mentioned excepted.) You say you beleeue not, and therefore drawe vppon you the payne due to the vnfaithfull: here beware deare brother, and waigh with circumspectipn, and due consideration

OF MELANCHOLIE.

tion of your state in so waightie a point as this is, and although you haue not at this time the sense thereof in your imagination, which is now disguised and blemished with melancholie conceits, and corporall alteration of the instrument of the bodie, yet do you beleeue, and shall hereafter feele the sweete comfort thereof, as you nowe aboundantly declare the fruites of so holy a roote; patience, meeknesse, charity, prayer, newnesse of life, and what soeuer good vertue springeth in the children of God therefrom. For euen as in outwarde senses we do see sometimes and feele, and heare; when wee do not perceaue it, so we may also haue faith, and not alwayes haue the sensible perceauing thereof; especiallie our bodies (as yours presently is) being oppressed with melancholie, which alwayes vrgeth terror and distrust: and deludeth vs with opinion of want of that, whereof wee haue no lacke: euen as in another extremitie, other men are oft carried with an opinion and confidence of those thinges whereof they haue no part. And if it be so with melancholickes, (as it is crediblie recorded in historie) that some haue complained they haue bene headlesse, so that (as Aëtius reporteth) Phylotymus the Phisitian was faine to put a cap of lead, vpon a melancholickes heade, that he might by feeing the waight conceaue otherwise; and Artenidorus the Grammarian did imagine he waned both a hand and a legge, though he wanted neither, you are to lay aside this fancie, and to weigh the presence of the cause by the effectes

O iiij

which are most euident tokens of faith in you, and not to rest vppon your deluded conceites, which if you yeeld vnto, will perswade you in the ende, that you want both head and heart also, after it hath dispossessed you in part of the right vse of both: but you will say vnto me, do not men otherwise doubt of this point but vpon melancholie? Yes verely: and especially such as most hunger and thirst after righteousnesse, and are poore in spirit, and broken in hart: the rest of the world, (except some vengeance of God laye holde vppon them, or some horrible fact gnawe their wounded conscience,) passing their time in a blinde securitie, carelesse of God, and emptie of all sense and hope of a better life, or feare of that eternall destruction; passe their dayes, and finish their course, as the calfe passeth to the shambles not knowing their ende to be slaughter by the butchers knife. Such I saye as are most carefull to walke before their God in righteousnesse, as they doubt and feare in euerie action, lest God be dishonoured by their conuersatiō, so are they ielouse of their pretious faith, lest it be not in such measure as they desire, or in truth be none at all: wherein they may easily be deceaued; first in the discerning, then in the measure and portion. Touching the discerning thus may they be ouertaken: when the inward feeling thereof doth not aunswere their desire, and the actions proceeding therfrom do not satisfie their thirst of righteousnesse, whereby reliefe may rise to the nourishment of faith, & the satisfying of that holy appetite; they are discouraged,

OF MELANCHOLIE.

couraged, and entangled with spirituall cares, from which a more aduised consideration agreable to Gods worde might easily deliuer them. Touching the portion, their fault lyeth in this, that they measure the excellencie thereof and the power, partly by measure, and quantitie, and not by vertue, wherewith through Gods mercifull grace it is indued to the saluation of all those that haue it but in measure of a graine of mustard seede: which both errours are to be corrected, by pondering of the case, not by that we iudge, but by that God him selfe hath geuen rule of: both touching the sense of faith, the sinceritie of the fruites, and increase of measure: all being his giftes and graces dispenced vnto vs, according to his mercie and wisedome, as is most for his glorie, and expedient for vs. For if we duly weigh from whence we are fallen, and howe deepe into this degenerate nature wherein we are captiues of Sathan, and slaues of all iniquitie, we shall receaue comfort of the least sparke of faith, and may praise God, and receaue comfort in the smallest worke of obedience perfourmed in sinceritie, though not in perfection: and if we finde the increases slowe, and the victorie harde in this our warfare: let vs consider with whome we fight, and for what crowne: and howe both heauen and earth was moued at our redemption: and the same power concurred thereto, as in our first creation. And as the great and mightie oakes are slower in attaining their full grouth, then shrubs and weedes, whose enduring is for many ages,

when' the other in short time wither and fadde away, so esteeme your encrease of heauenly graces slow, but sure, euerlasting as immortalitye, that you may be as a beame or a piller in the tēple of God for euer and euer. Neither are we to accompt the nature of any thing according to our sense or to the shew it maketh. For then should the most fruitefull tree in winter be takē for barren, and the lustie soile dry, and vnfruitefull while it is shut vp with the hard frost: but reason (as in other deliberatiōs) so in this must lead vs (being guided by the word of God) rightly to iudge of the presence, & life of faith in our souls: which being the shield in this our spirituall warfaire, endureth much battering & many bruntes and receiueth the forefront of the encounter, & oft times faireth as if it were pearced through and worne, vnfit for battaile: yet is it in deede of nature inuincible, and repelleth whatsoeuer ingine the enimy inforceth against vs, and stādeth firme rooted: whatsoeuer storme Sathan raiseth for the displacing thereof. How then are we to behaue our selues in this temptation: whē both the sence of faith is dulled in vs, and the fruites minister discontentment? you remember the saying of the Apostle, the graces and mercy of God is without repentance, and Christ Iesus whome he loueth, to the end he loueth them: if then you haue in times past felt that gift of the spirit, (which you haue done) & haue ioyed therin: be assured it is a marke neuer to be defaced, of your election & firme stāding in Gods fauour. For what moued the Lord to bestow the grace:
but

but his owne mercy:& that he bestoweth:who cā take away if he himselfe take it frō vs,for some deserte of ours,did not he foresee the same lōg before ? & so why did he not withold his mercy?but as he knew vs when we were straungers from him,and loued vs,when we hated him, and had nothing which might prouoke his mercy, but our misery:so is his goodnes continued vpon vs still for his owne sake, and not at all for our deseruing: that all being subiect to his condemnation, he might be glorified in the saluation of some, for that righteousnes sake which is in his sonne, and that oblation of his offered vp, not for himselfe but for others: from whose righteousnes so much is detracted as we attribute vnto our selues,or seeke to attaine vnto, in respect of satisfying Gods iustice:and so much impaired of Gods mercy,as we shall rest vpon any vertue or power in our selues, whereby to auoid his végeance of iustice: Our election as it first riseth from God, and is established in his immutable counsell and decree, and lyeth in no power else beside: so the hazard thereof is not committed to the aduenture of our frailty, but the continuance and stablenes in the same decree hath the foūdation. For alas the wofull experience of Adams frailty in his best estate giueth sufficient testimony,and more then sufficient: what hope there is of continuance of grace, if the assurāce of our saluation should depend vpon our keeper who without support of God are like the wynde inconstant and as fraile as the tender hearbs, and want all habilitie of withstāding the assaults

of our enimie: and constant perseuerance in any religious vertue, and worke of pietie. Then if the foundation of our election lie in the counsell of God, and be founded vpon his decree: who hath reuealed the one but the Spirit of the Lord, and what is able to vndermine the other where the Lord himselfe hath layed the corner stone? This assurance in time past the Spirite of God hath confirmed vnto you, & you haue felt it with plēty of heauenly ioy, and comfort: and if in the cōflict of temptation you esteeme the strength according to that remaineth after the battaile, or that which you feele being somewhat tyred in the conflict: you may here giue vauntage to the ennemy through discouragement, and loose the field as much as lieth in you, wher there is hope of assured victory. For, be it that you feele the hability weake, and the ennemy strong, and your owne corruption vpon the point to preuaile, yet consider there is a roote of this vertue, whose fruite, and braunches although these stormy tēpestes may nippe and shake, yet the sappe shall neuer be dried vp in the roote, neither can anie euill winde of Sathan so blast, that the immortall seed be at any time quit withered, yea though all his fiery dartes be thereto with all might and maine employed, but that the storme being blone ouer by the spirite of grace, and the comfortable sunne of consolation shining vpon our gloumie heartes, it will budde forth againe into blossome, fruit, and braunch, as a most beautifull tree in the paradice of God. Let the comparison of bodely sicknes, and the consideration of that
kinde

Of Melancholie.

kinde of frailty, giue comforte vnto you in your case although in an other kinde, yet in this respect not vnlike. We haue experiéce how diuerse times the deseafe preuaileth ouer the ficke persons, that actiuns faile and faculties seeme quite to be spent, neither hand nor foote is able to do their duetie, the eye is dimme, the hearing dull, the tast altered, and the tounge diftafteth all things euē of most pleasant relish, and the weak and feeble pacient seemeth to attend the time of dissolution: when yet notwithstanding there remaineth a secret power of nature, and a forcible spark of life that ouercōmeth all these infirmities, and consumeth them like drosse, & rendereth to the body a greater purity, & firmenes of health then before the sicknes it did enioy. Euen so esteeme of the spirituall case, and consider that your soule is sicke and not dead, and faith is assailed but not ouercome, & only haue patience to attend the finishing of this secret worke which passeth all conceite, and capacity of man, and you shall see these burning feauers, of temptations to be slaked and cooled by the mercy and grace of Christ, and that sparke of faith which lieth now hidde, and ouerwhelmed with heapes of temptation, and seemeth to be vtterly quenched to breake forth againe, and to consume these straunge causes of the deseafe of the soule, and as nature after a perfect crise dischargeth her self either by stoole, vomite, sweat, or bleeding, or such like euacuations, to the recouerie of former health, so shall you feele all these doubtes, and feares, and terrors remoued, and strength of faith restored with such supply, as it shallbe able to make euident proofe what secrete vertue laye hid and yet not idle in all this vncomfortable plight which offereth you temptation of dispaire. Seing then that you are yet but vnder the conflict: and not ouercome, haue good cheare in the succession which as in Christ it is victorious, ouer head; so are we (his partes & members,) to looke for the same crowne of glory, who both ouercome in him, & through him, in our selues shall in the ende be possessed of the victory, and receiue the crowne of immortality. As for that which your owne conceit corrupted by melancholy perswadeth you, & wherin Sathan is busie, and omitteth no oportunity: giue no credite thereunto, but as it is, so esteeme it a delusion which time will discouer and lay open, as you your selfe shall hereafter most planly discerne. I graunt you, the temptation it selfe though your body were free from this infirmity, is of the greatest kinde, & such as doth not skirmish only lightly vpon our soules, but setteth the maine battaile against our most happy estate, in so much as it forced our Sauiour to cry, my God my God, why hast thou forsaken me. But what then? are we therefore to be discouraged? no, no, here appeareth rather the aboundance of Gods grace, and the mightie supporte of his power, which euen in the middest of hel preserueth his and suffereth not so much as their garments to take any smell of the flame, but euen from thece is able to raise them to his celestiall kingdome & place, them which his sonne in the throne of

glory

glory. And if you dewly consider the price of our redemption how pretious it was, & how it could not be obtayned, without shedding of the most pretious heartblood of the sonne of God, you must thinke the quarrell to be no other to the ende, but a matter of blood, of strife, of sweate, of feare, of ielousie, and whatsoeuer affection goeth with affecting a glorious triumph in all the mēbers of Christ, both inwardly and outwardly, in the spirite and in the body, as our head himselfe could finde in dispensation though he sued vnto his father therefrom with aboundance of tears: and thinke that it is Gods busines we are in hād with, and that we are inabled of him, and accōpt not these smal venies of Satā for deadly woūdes which are no thing other but practises, and exercises of the spirituall courage, and circumspection, and introductions to that vse of the whole armour of God, where against no force of the enemy shall preuaile, though the attempt seeme to be full of perill, & terror. But you say you feele small strength of faith, & no support of that hope which maketh not ashamed. Beware least you iudge vniustly of the wayes of God, & esteeme that for small which is great, and vile which in the sight of God is most pretious. For herein the ennemy may take encouragement to your great disaduantage. You feele not that taste thereof you sometimes felt: and do you iudge therefore you are bereued vtterly thereof? what? consider the soule is now sick, & disteftacth much wholesome meate of consolation, and loatheth many pleasaunt and fragraunt cuppes of comfort, and counsell, and yet the indeuours of Gods childre in this behalfe, and the sweete waters of heauēly comfort are not therefore of themselues bitter or vnsauory, so you are not to measure the absence of this grace by that you presently, but by that in times past (while the soule stoode free from this disease of tēptation, & trial) you haue felt of comfort in the spirite through an acceptable measure of faith according to the dispensation of Gods grace, and not according to our fancy, but as he shal think meete to be ministred vnto vs. Neither is the tryall of faith only to be taken according as the soule feeleth it in it selfe but also and sometimes (as in such temptations as these wherein you now trauaile) onely by the course and trade of life which hath passed before, and those fruites which are euident to the eye of others who can iudge more sincerely then the afflicted whose vnderstandinges are somewhat altered through Sathans terrors. But againe you say the course of life past, and your estate present hath nothing aunswered the holines of your vocation, and that sinceritie the Lord requireth so that here also the comforte faileth you. What then? are you therfore reprobate? No, but it argueth want of faith, not so, but place for farther increase of faith and the fruits thereof. Those whome the Lord hath chosen to be his worshipers, and hath redeemed, and consecrated holy to himselfe, and prepared good workes for them to walke in: they be his plantes and ingraffed oliue braūches in his sonne which take not their full perfection at once, but according glorie. And if you duly consider the price of our redemption how pretious it was, & how it could not be obtained, without shedding of the most pretious hart bloud of the Sonne of God: you must thinke the quarrell to be no other to the ende, but a matter of bloud, of strife, of sweate, of feare, of ielousie, and whatsoeuer affection goeth with affecting a glorious triumph in all the members of Christ: both inwardly, and outwardly, in the spirit and in the bodie: as our head himselfe could finde no dispensation, though he sued vnto his Father therfore with aboundance of teares: and thinke that it is Gods businesse we are in hand with, & that we are inabled of him, mooued and carried by his spirite, increase with his increases, not to be measured with the eye of flesh, or carnall vnderstanding, but by the same spirite which worketh in vs: who as he hath begunne, will also make perfect his worke to his owne glory: which lieth in taking pity and compassion, more aboundantly then in shewing végeance. By this which hitherto hath bene said, it appeareth plainly that no sinne hath yet passed you, which can seclude you from hope of saluation; and therefore necessarily it followeth that the crosse you are now vnder is an attempt of Satan against you, to cast you into vtter dispaire and if it were possible to vndoe that knot more surely knit then that of Gordius, which coupleth vs vnto our God, and wherewith we are espoused vnto Iesus Christ: euen our most glorious faith which ouercommeth the world: & where against not Satā, nor all his force, or stratageme

P

is able to preuaile. I say it is only a temptation of the ennemy purposed of him to your confusion: but from your louing God, and mercifull father, a triall of faith and patience, and the proofe of those vertues which before laye hid in secrete: which he will haue now shew themselues in the combat, he himselfe a beholder, an incourager, a succour at neede, and prest with the crowne of triumph to giue rewarde, and honour to the victory. Wherefore, only haue patience: be not discouraged: stand sure, and the feeblenes of Sathan shall soone appeare: and his weapons shall be al broaken in peeces, and God (through faith and patience, and comfort of the Scriptures by his spirite) shall be glorified in the weakenes of his poore afflicted seruant: and you shall againe (as Dauid was) be restored to those wōted ioyes which you haue sometimes felt in the sweete mercies of the Lord. Now the ground of all tēptation is our owne weakenes, this is tried and proued by Sathan or the world, or both ioyned together as considerations of our destruction. Besides this continual buddes of iniquity which do rise from our originall corruption, Sathan sometimes playeth his part vpon our weakenes alone, and sometimes by outward temptations, and sometimes layeth siege round about vs, and besetteth all the parts of our complete armour. We are weake in vnderstanding and in whatso euer action riseth therefrom; euen in will & affection: Our vnderstanding is turned into blindnes of error; Our will embraceth not only those thinges which corrupt iudgement directeth vnto,

Of Melancholie.

to, but euen wher sometime vnderstanding stãdeth sound, ther will bēdeth to affection, & neglecteth the light of reason. Our affections are both rebellious to right iudgement and will: in that they rage where they should not, and wher iust cause is giuen there they inordinately exceed. Thus iudgement, wil, and affection, hauing degenerated, vse the bodely members as weapons and instrumentes of all impietye, and in iustice: so that if the grace of God did not for preseruation of humaine society, and especially for his Churches cause restraine this strēgth of iniquity, the pillers of the world would shatter in sunder, and the vault of heauen would fall, & all things woulde turne againe to their former Chaos, & be consumed with the terrible fire of Gods vengeaunce, and perishe in his heauy displeasure. Our misery being such, no maruaile though both Sathan and the world preuaile against vs, except the Lord stretch foorth his hand, and vphold vs. This our infirmity Sathan doth sometimes assaye without meanes: and sometimes by outward occasions of euill, & forcible perswasion of sinne, and rebelliō against God. How he doth it without means, the experience is more lamentable and infallible, then the manner how easie to finde out. In corporall possession it seemeth there needeth no meanes: when Sathan possesseth all partes of the howse, and as maister commaundeth at his pleasure. But how without such accesse he is able to tēpt, that is a matter of more difficult consideration: which, because it maketh not a litle to the bet-

P ij

ter laying open of your estate, I will somewhat stande vpon: referring you for the rest to the resolutions of the diuines who haue chiefe part in this busines. For my owne part I do take it, & am assured you find the experience, that Sathā after a personall manner vnto the soule, though not in bodely shape to the eye, without meanes of outward thinges which (might moue our wils or affections) tempteth vs in the very secrete thoughts of our heartes. For being a spirite, and by creation most excellent, it is not to be doubted but that he hath a spirituall accesse vnto our spirites, to trouble them, and to disorder all their actions, as we see corporall creatures, with bodely and corporall force, to annoy one an other. And as men haue fellowship one with other by corporall presence, and are delighted or displeased with the quallities of the minde according as they like, or dislike, vttered by speach & talke: so is it most like that the spirites haue their society maintained by a spirituall conference, whereby their wills and purposes are entercommunicated one to an other, without corporall sound, whereof both the spirites want the instrument, and the voice nothing affecteth the mind. Dayly experience maketh this manifest in such as are possessed, how Sathan so beareth the sway in them that their speach and phrase altereth, and their discourse is farre other then before, & their whole nature at Sathans becke, and their vtterance of minde as he only suggesteth. In others whome Sathan hath not layed such hold on, the same no lesse is to be seene: as when the

false

OF MELANCHOLIE.

false prophetes did deceiue Ahab: there came forth a spirit which was sent to be a false & lying spirite in the mouth of all his prophets, which accordingly did make promis vnto him of victory, who notwithstāding found a contrary euent of ouerthrow,& destructiō. So entred Satan into Iudas the traitor,& moued him to betray our Sauiour, not by a corporall possession: but by a spirituall impulsion whereby he worketh in the children of disobedience, and Peter in the fift of the Actes sayeth to Ananias: why hath Sathan filled thine heart,&c: and againe in the second to the Ephesians the Apostle calleth the Deuill the prince that ruleth in the ayre, the spirite that nowe worketh in the children of disobedience: by which it is plaine that the deuill hath power where God permitteth him ouer the minds and iudgements, and wills of the reprobate, and wicked: and may also in such sort tempt the faithful seruants of God. For the Apostle saith in the same place, that the Ephesians (to whome he wrote) in times past walked according to the course of this world,& after the conduct of that spirite. Neither do we stande thus subiect vnto Sathans annoyance through the subtlenesse of his nature, being a spirit; but through that lōg experience and practise of our miserie from age to age, whereby he is able with ease to worke our anoyance in all respects. This giueth him knowledge of our mindes more perfectly: who apprehendeth the same by the least shew, and inclination of our affection & wil. Not that he knoweth our harts, entirely and perfectly: which is proper to God only the framer of the hart, but only through that triall and experience which not one onely particular man hath miniſtred vnto him, but euen our whole race from Adam to this preſent: this maketh him not to expect anie outward ſignification of ſpeach, or geſture, to conceiue our intents and purpoſes: but out of our vniuerſall corruption whereof he hath continuall prooſe, he hath layed vp matter of argument to diſcouer the vanity of our mindes, and the ſecret thoughtes of our heart: which after he hath found, he ſuggeſteth (as he ſeeth occaſion wherto we muſt incline) inſtigation of ſinne & diſobedience againſt God, & his holy commandemēts. His temptatiōs are properly ſuch, as neither our natures ſeme to incline vnto, but in a generality to all kinde of wickednes; nor the world doth either allure vs, or inforce vs: eſpecially the children of god who are partakers of his ſpirit finde them moſt ſtraunge, and ſuch as they abhorre the very leaſt conceite of them, & finde no parte of their nature to incline vnto them, howſoeuer in other reſpectes they complaine of frailty. Of this kinde are ceitaine blaſphemies ſuggeſted of the Deuill, and laying of violent handes of them ſelues, or vpon others neither moued therto by hate or malice: or any occaſion of reuenge: of the ſame ſort is the diſpaire and diſtruſt of gods mercy, and grace, beſides many other as taking away the ſeede of the word out of the heart of the negligent hearers: the ſuggeſting of errors & ſuch like without our natures ſpeciall inclination that way, but rather contrarily affected. And

as

as he is a spirite, & an effectuall worker in other meanes: so when he applieth his proper trauaile he attempteth the most daungerous assaults, to our saluation: and entereth so deep that (knowing the iudgement is the fountaine of all vertuous action) there he maketh traine, and after a spirituall manner seeketh possession thereof to the vtter descouraging of all your actions that depend thereon: knowing that it once being at his deuotion, the corporall grosse actions & bodely vices, neede no great prouocation. Other temptations rise of our owne rebellious heartes vnto the holy commandementes of God: or frō the wordely allurements, which as baites entice vs frō the way of obedience: or else from terrors of life which scar vs with threate of perill, if we embrace the way of piety, and of holines: and setteth before vs a greater awe of men, then we haue of feare, & reuerence of God. Now among these temptations falleth your present estate, & especially Sathan employeth his force to your iudgement, and not against the strength of carnall iudgement only, but against that which the Spirite of God hath taught and sealed vnto you in your conscience: both suggesting vnto you those blasphemous conceites which your heart ytterly abhorreth the least thought and remembrāce of, and raiseth that doubt of Gods fauour which now diuersly distracteth you. Remember I pray you, how the spirite of God calleth him the tempter, the deceiuer of the world: and the accuser of the faithfull: the Dragon and old serpent, a lyer, and the father of lies: by which epethites, and descriptions, you may consider his power, his malice, and his craft to deceaue, and to abuse you: neuer before acquainted with his practises as at this present you haue experience of: and not take all that your minde conceiueth of any manner of impiety whatsoeuer, to be from you, but from Sathan: who as he hath power to tempt and to trie, to cast before you these stumbling blockes whereat he would haue you fall:so hath he no power to fasten them vpō your minde, and to giue them setteling: your owne conscience bearing you witnes how much repugnant they are to your desires. The rather are you to accompt thē as frō him, because they be such, as are altogether cōtrary to your former conuersation, & whereto you haue felt your nature incline before, and such as haue no inforcement nor inticemēt from any creature, but from him. Wherefore though such kinde of thoughts doe assaile the hart, that (being guilty of so great sinne) your cōsciēce might be so much the more defiled, and the discouragement the greater; yet aunswere them againe by the word of God which is the sworde of the spirite: and wayte the happie ende of the conflict with patience: and accompt not these small venies of Sathan for deadly wounds, which are nothing else but practises, & exercises of your spirituall courage, & circumspection: & introductions to that vse of the whole armour of God, where against no force of the enemie shall preuaile, though the attempt seeme to be full of perill, and terrour. But you say you feele small strength of faith, and

no

no support of that hope which maketh not ashamed. Beware least you iudge vniustly of the wayes of God, and esteeme that for small which is great, and vile, which in the sight of God is most pretious. For herein the enemie may take encouragement, to your great disaduauntage. You feele not that taste thereof you sometimes felt: and do you iudge therefore you are bereued vtterlie thereof? what? consider the soule is nowe sicke, and distasteth much wholesome meate of consolation, and loatheth many pleasaunt and fragrant cuppes of comfort, and counsell, and yet the indeuours of Gods childrē in this behalfe, and the sweete waters of heauēly comfort are not therefore of themselues bitter or vnsauory, so you are not to measure the absence of this grace by that you presently, but by that in times past (while the soule stoode free from this disease of tēptation, & trial) you haue felt of comfort in the spirite through an acceptable measure of faith according to the dispensation of Gods grace, and not according to our fancy, but as he shal think meete to be ministred vnto vs. Neither is the tryall of faith only to be taken according as the soule feeleth it in it selfe but also (and sometimes as in such temptations as these wherein you now trauaile onely) by the course and trade of life which hath passed before, and those fruites which are euident to the eye of others who can iudge more sincerely then the afflicted whose vnderstandinges are somewhat altered through Sathans terrors. But againe you say the course of life past, and your estate present hath nothing aunswered the holines of your vocation, and that sinceritie the Lord requireth so that here also the comforte faileth you. What then? are you therfore reprobate? No, but it argueth wāt of faith; Not so; but place for farther increase of faith, and the fruits thereof. Those whome the Lord hath chosen to be his worshipers, and hath redeemed, and consecrated holy to himselfe, and prepared good workes for them to walke in: they be his plantes and ingraffed oliue braūches in his sonne who take not their ful perfection at once (but according to the nature of a plāt) require dayly watering & dressing, wherby by degrees they attaine in the ende a full stature in Christ. So that you may not accompt your selfe voyde of grace, because you are not perfect (for in this life both faith, and knowledge, and loue are all imperfect, and shall partly be furnished, and partly receaue perfectiō elsewhere,) but you are godly & wisely to consider the secret worke of Gods spirite, and grace, and take comfort of the smallest crumme and drop of this heauenly sustentation and attend your time of perfect growth, according to the good pleasure of God. You can not at all times feele and followe with your conceit, and naturall capacitie the worker of this mysterie: more then you are able to discerne where the wind riseth; and where it lighteth. You know we that are called, are borne againe, and as the growth and increase of our bodies is not perceaued of vs, though we do increase, & the birth is not apprehended of the infant borne & bred,

euen

Of Melancholie.

euen so is it with vs in the heauenly birth, and spirituall regeneration, the spirit worketh without our leaue, and acquainteth vs not with his maruelous working more then is expedient at his pleasure, when, and in what measure for our comfort: much lesse can a body ouercharged with melancholy, & drowned in that darke dungeon see the comfortable beames of his day starre, & brightnesse of the cheerfull Sunne of God aboundant mercie, and a mind whose actions are hindered by meanes thereof, whereby it neither conceiueth nor iudgeth sincerely and vprightly as the case requireth: and neither so only affected, but blinde folded by the humour, and brought into this darknesse of feare, is buffited also and beaten with Sathan on all sides, whereby being distracted, it obtayneth no respit, and releale, of due and iust consideration, howe can it discerne rightly of these thinges? Wherefore your case being such, yeelde not so much to the enemy, as to iudge of your selfe according to his sentence, who is a lyer from the beginning, and the father of lyes; but according to those olde testimonies which you haue felt in your owne conscience, and haue giuen comfortable shewe of to others in the course of your life heretofore. Oh, but you feele not the testimonie of Gods spirit, which might assure you. Neither do any of Gods children at all times feele it. Dauid cōplained of the want hereof; Iob complained likewise, & so haue diuerse of Gods children in all times made mone hereof. Sufficient it is if at any time that assurance be giuen,

and if it be the will of God for a time to withdraw it, that you may feeling your owne frailty, with more earnest desire call to him for his wonted grace: Who are you to interrupt the wayes of God, and to preuent his counselles? and for your comfort be assured that the former grace, you haue receaued is of that nature, that it neuer decayeth, but remaineth an euerlasting seed of immortalitie, procceding from the Father of eternitie, and with whom there is no chaungeablenesse, nor shadowe of turning: who doth nothing to repent him of, but is only wise, stable, & sure, and hath no neede to correct anie thing of his owne workmanship. And if he withhold the comfort of his spirite from you for a season, it is that you may with greater appetite seeke after it, and hauing found it, more ioy therein, and praise his mercie with thankfulnesse of hart, and readinesse of vtterance to sound out the aboundance of his mercie. If the Lord withhold it not, but the frailtie wherein you stand, diminish the sense thereof, or the temptation presse so farre vpon you that you are not free to iudge aright, or the perill which the temptation carieth with it moue you to distrust, knowe that nothing befalleth you straunge herein more then to other of Gods children before you, and that to wade through these violent streames, patience and constancie is most needfull, with a resolute mind to abide the Lords wil, who in the end wil come, and will not tarie. This is the broken & contrite heart which the Lord will not despise, this is the poore spirit, on whome the Lord pronounceth
bles-

blessednesse, and this is the affliction whereof the Spirit of God is called the comforter: so that (although before the Lord hath vouchsafed you many graces,) yet were you neuer meete to receaue diuerse other which he will nowe bestowe vpon you, before this present: and so shall you in the end receaue the cup of saluation in steed of the bottell of vineger and teares, and in steed of the bread of affliction the heauenly Manna, and the bread of life from the table of God & Christ. Wherefore suspect these thoughtes to be of the enemie and not of your selfe, cast into your mind of him, and not springing of incredulitie: I am out of Gods fauour: I am reprobate from his kingdome, there remaineth no hope for me: I haue no faith. For such are his temptations of old, & daily they be the points he laboureth in against Gods childré, if not to wring fró thé their hope, at the least to weary their dayes with heauinesse, and discomfort. Neither esteeme your selfe, presently by that you feele; but by that you haue felt, when nothing hath ouershadowed that light of knowledge, faith, and zeale, but the full brightnesse of these graces hath broken forth. For why haue not these doubts risen vnto you before time? and where is nowe the auncient assurance? They before time rose not, because the temptation was far of, and that assurance although by tempest of temptation, and by this spirituall storme it seeme to bend, and to giue backe, yet is it inuincible, and recouereth thereby more strength then euer it had before. Is the souldier worse appayed that sustaineth the combat, and standeth in the face of his enemie, though the terrible thunder of shot beat his eares, and he in perill of hitting; though he maintaine the heate of the battell against the force of his enemie with perill? not a whit: he becommeth hereby more valiant: he learneth experience, his skill increaseth, and his courage doubleth vppon him. So in this spirituall battaile you must not be discouraged like a milk soppe, or a fresh souldier vntrained or vnacquainted with warfare: but set the victorie before your eyes, which is alreadie attained and purchased for you: and so much the more are you to endure with Christian valiance, in that here is no feare of ouerthrowe: the battaile is broken, and the enemies scattered, and onely the captaine requireth to be followed of you for whome he hath obtained the crowne of victorie, if the stragling tayle of the enemie annoye they may shewe their malice and hostilitie but their force is foyled; and take heart onely, and endure, and you shall see them vanquished, and submit vnto that power of Christ which inableth you. You must consider that as in warfare the seruice is not alwayes alike, neither keepeth the souldier the same degree, but is aduaunced of the generall as he seeth cause: euen so if the Lorde nowe bestowe you in a straunge peece of seruice in his spirituall warre, and place you in the forefront, whome he hath hitherto rendered as your condition required, you must be contented, and quite your selfe like a man, and knowe that the wisedome of

the

the heauenly captaine is such, and his tender affection so great towarde his followers, that in the middest of perill, not one haire of them shall miscarrie whom he leadeth. Then to conclude this point, seing your case is onely a téptation, and no temptation is of it selfe (except that one) a signe of reprobation: cast of these discouragementes: and learne howe to behaue your selfe herein, that you may passe through with credit of your vocation, and honour vnto God, & ioy & comfort to your faithful friends in the Lord Iesus. You haue read your selfe & may partly perceaue by my former discourse howe melancholie perswadeth of miserie where there is no cause, & some haue imagined themselues to haue wanted their heads, some their armes, other some haue thought themselues dead men, and other some one member of their bodies as bigge as three: which as it perswadeth in corporal things that which is not, so no lesse doth it in spirituall things especially, being like a weapó taken into Sathans hand, and vsed to all aduantages of our hurt and destruction. This maketh all more grieuous, & is called of Serapio, the very seate of the deuill being an apt instrument for him, both to weaken our bodies with, and to terrifie our minds with vaine, & fantasticall feares, and to disturbe the whole tranquillity of our nature. Wherefore ascribe I pray you these troubles of your mind to no other, but to the frailty of your bodie: I meane this excesse of distrust, & feare, otherwise the temptation may be without it: and giue no way to Sathans practise, in yeelding your iudgement and affection to his suggestion; but resist as against a sicknesse, and as nature doth with her spirit against bodily disease, so take courage, and call together the wisdome, and knowledge God hath giuen you, and nowe put it in vse against this subtle, and forcible enemie. And through Gods blessing by due vse of such naturall means as I shall hereafter declare vnto you, both mind and bodie shall againe be restored to the former integritie, and you haue greater cause then euer to prayse God for his niercie, and goodnesse towardes you. Hitherto nothing hath befallen you, that diuerse of Gods children haue not passed through before you, & although the battaile hath bene sharp & bloudy euen as our Maister hath sweat dropps of bloud in the like combat, remember the victorie is the more glorious, and the conquest so much the more honorable & sure: as we haue experience in the person of Iesus our Sauiour which found no other way to his kingdome, and hath left vnto vs an example of like patience, constancie, & hope, and whatsoeuer vertue else is requisite to this battaile of the spirit, and doth furnish vs in all partes with spirituall armour. He girdeth vs with truth, and buckleth on vs the brestplate of righteousnesse: he shoeth our feet with the preparation of the Gospell of peace: he deliuereth into the left hand the shield of faith, wherby we may quench the firie dartes of the deuill, & into the right, the sword of the spirite, the word of God, and couereth our heads with the helmet of saluation. If we shall cowardly cast our armor

and

Of Melancholie.

and weapon from vs, and betake vs to flight, besides there is no place of safetie, we shall dishonour our captaine, giue ouer our selues to the pleasure and crueltie of our enemie, and finally perish for euer. Wherefore trie the strength of this armour, and the sharpnesse of this sword, & nowe occasion is offered, march on with those shoes of peace, which is the ende of warre, and wherof they are the pledge and assurance, hold out that shield of faith, and although it be battered on all sides, yet forsake it not, for the temper is such as no fierie darte of the wicked can pierce it: and bestowe that sword of Gods word, the word of consolation, of ioy, of assurance, of spirituall and heauenly wisedome, whereby the iudgement is perfected, & the hart established, and the whole man of God made absolute. Forsake not that breastplate of the righteousnesse of Iesus Christ, and that frute of our sanctification whereby we are in his Sonne acceptable vnto God: & with the helmet of saluation couer your head, that all the good meanes of God being to the full employed, you may feele the power of this heauenly furniture to your present encouragement, & herafter to your euerlasting saluation. Let not your sinnes dismay you, for Christ came not to saue the righteous, he supplieth all our wantes, and hath aboundance to discharge our debtes. In him is God well pleased with vs, as himselfe hath pronounced, so that being discharged in him, let vs giue ouer all feare, & with boldnes approch vnto the throne of grace that we may receaue the mercie promised vnto vs,

Q

for if we be righteouse, then is Christ vnrighteous, and suffered for him selfe, and not for vs: but he was iust & pure, a lambe without spot or blemish slaine for the attonemēt, that we might thereby liue, broaken that we might be healed, and humbled for our aduancement. Wherefore lay the burthen vpon him, who hath sayd, come vnto me all ye that are heauy loden, and he shall ease your wearied shoulders thereof, and geue you refreshing. If ther were no sinne wheron should Gods mercie be shewen? and whereto tendeth the promise of the Gospell? But you say you are a great sinner: what then? is not the mercie of God greater? is there anie ende of his compassion? If sinne do abound, who shall stint the grace of God, that it should not also ouerflow? Dauid was a great sinner, so was both Peter and Paule: yet were they not refused, but receaued mercie. And if the grace of God were so great, that our sinnes could not withholde his mercie when we were straungers from his couenant, aliens from the common wealth of Israell, and led with that spirit of errour, and darknesse, like the nations that knowe not God; much more being reconciled, stand we sure, and vnremoueable in his fauour, though the cloudes do somtimes ouercast the bright beames therof, & our owne imbecillitie comprehendeth it not. Remember the tryall of Iob: who would haue taken him for other, then one forsaken of the Lord? what were his thoughts? let the day perish wherin I was borne. Why died I not in the birth? wherefore is light giuen vnto him that is in misery,

Of Melancholie.

fery, and life vnto them that haue heauy harts? And in an other place: oh that I were as in times past! when God preserued me, whē his light shined vpon my head, &c. But what was the tryall? God blessed the last dayes of Iob more thē the first: euen so, though the present afflictiō be grieuous vnto you, and all hope faile in respect of your feeling, yet the Lord when he hath proued you and found you his pure and sincere beloued sonne, the like issue are you assured of with comforte in this life, and eternall saluation in the life to come. Thus leauing a more plentifull consolation vnto your godly friendes who dayly frequent you, especially such as are preachers of the word and ministers of Gods grace, I proceed to instruct you in that I iudge your body stādeth in neede of, that howsoeuer hability faile in performāce of the offices of friendships on my part, towards you, my sincere affection and vnfayned loue vnto you may be at the least testified by my endeuour: wherein if I be tedious partly it is of forgetfulnes of that consideration, being ouercaried with desire to benefite you, and partly bicause in your case I also comprehend the estate of many one at this day in like sort affected and afflicted, who if they receiue any meanes of cōforte by this my trauaile, they may be more beholding vnto my friēd M. & pray for his release. Thus my good M. you haue the testimonie of my good will in this part of counsell. I confesse I am not so meet for it, as your case requireth: but so haue I discharged that office wherto the dutie of friendship bindeth me. If my presence may supply the defect, I will not faile you wherein anie part of mine abilitie may serue your wāts I will nowe proceede to the cure of your bodie, whose disorder increaseth your heauinesse, and ioyneth hand with this kind of temptation.

Chap. XXXVII.
The cure of melancholy, and howe melancholicke persons are to order them selues in actions of the mind, sense, and motion.

AS the ordinarie cure of all diseases, & helps of infirmities are to be begun with remouing of such causes as first procured the infirmitie (except they be remoued of them selues, through their nature, neither stable nor permanent) by succession of a contrarie cause of the same kinde: euen so the first entry of restoring the melancholicke braine and heart, to a better state of conceit, and cheere, is the remouing of such causes as first disturbed iudgement, and affection, or are therto apt, with inducing of causes of contrarie operation. The causes of all diseases are either breach of dutie, and some errour cōmitted in the gouernment of our health; or such accidentes as befall vs in this life against our wills, and vnlooked for. From the same also do arise the workes of melancholie, whereof I intreate, and you desire to be released. Our diet consisteth not onely (as it is commonly taken) in meate, and drinke: but in whatsoeuer exercises of mind or bodie: whether they be studies of the braine, or affections of the hart, or whether
they

they be labours of the bodies, or exercises only. Besides vnto diet, house, habitation, and apparel do belong, which are causes of maintenance, or ouerthrowe of health, as they be affected. To these also the order of rest, and sleepe is to be added as a great meanes, taken in due time, and in conuenient moderation, to preserue health, or to cause sicknesse, if otherwise it be taken immoderatly, too scant, or disorderly. Of the labours of the mind, studies haue great force to procure melancholie: if they be vehement, and of difficult matters, and high misteries: & therfore chiefly they are to be auoyded, & the mind to be set free from all such trauel, that the spirits which before were partly wasted, might be restored: and partly employed vpon hard discourses, may be released, to the comfort of the hart, and thinning of the bloud. Besides, such actions approching nigh vnto, or being the verie inorganicall of the soule, cause the mind to neglect the bodie: whereby easily it becmometh afterward vnapt for the action, and the humours skanted of the sweet influence thereof, and spirit, setle into a melancholie thicknesse, and congele into that cold and drie humour, which rayseth these terrours and discouragements. Wherfore aboue all, abandon working of your braine by any studie, or conceit: and giue your mind to libertie of recreation, from such actions, that drawe too much of the spirit, and therby wrong the corporall mēbers of the bodie. For in maintainance of health it is specially to be obserued, that the employing of the parts either of mind or bodie with their spirite, is to be carried with such indifferencie, and discretion, that the force which should be common to manie, be not lauishly spent vpon any one. Nowe, studie, of all actions, both because it vseth litle help of the bodie, in comparison of other: and because the minde chieflie laboureth, which draweth the whole bodie into sympathie, wherby it is neglected as it were for a time, and the most subtile & purest spirits thereby are consumed, is to be giuen ouer in the cure of this passion: or if the affection can not be tempered wholly therefrom, then such matter of studie is to be made choyse of, as requireth no great contention, but with a certaine mediocritie, may vnbend that stresse of the minde, through that ouer vehement action, and withall carie a contentednesse thereto, and ioy to the affection. Nowe as all contention of the mind is to be intermitted, so especially that, whereto the melancholicke person most hath giuen him selfe before the passion is chieflie to be eschued, for the recouerie of former estate, and restoring the depraued conceit, and fearefull affection. For there, if the affection of liking go withall, both hart, and braine do ouer prodigally spend their spirits, and with them the subtilest partes of the naturall iuyce, and humours of the bodie. If of mislike, and the thing be by forcible constraint layd on, the distracting of the mind, from the promptnes of the affection breedeth such an agonie in our nature, that thereon riseth also great expeence of spirit, and of the most rare and subtile humours of our bodies, which

which are as it were the seate of our naturall heate, the refiner of all our humours, and the purifier of our spirites. As that kind of studie, wherein the melancholicke hath spent him selfe is to be auoyded, or intermitted, and one of a milder and softer kinde to be inferred in place thereof, so much lesse anie straunge studie of difficultie, and much trauell of the braine is to be taken in hand, as it were to turne the minde into a contrarie bent. For herein the straungenesse, besides difficultie giueth cause of trauaile and toile vnto our nature: so that both these extremities are to be eschued of you as most daungerous, and hurtfull, and the mind to be retired to such a tranquillitie, as the naturall heate and spirits may haue free scope to attend vppon the corporall actions of preparing the bloud, and thinning of the grosse iuice into a moderate substance, as is according to good disposition of the bodie. In studie I comprehend (although they be diuerse) all action of internall senses, which are ministers and seruants of studie, whether it be of learning, or of meditation, and inuention: which later kind, farre more toyleth the bodie, then the former, and therefore farther of is it to be remoued. Of internall senses, I take phantasie to be the greatest wast of these spirits, & most apt to thicken the bloud, if it be excessiue. For that imitateth the inuentiue action of the mind, and in a lower degree (if it be vehement & continuall) maketh great wast of those two instruments, spirit, and heate, in the melancholicke bodie. For as the action is, such is the spirit, and part thereof purer, subtiler, thinner, as the actiõ is of more excellency, & farther remoued from corporall practise, and draweth nigher to the cleere, and pure actions of the minde. If the melancholicke be ouer much contemplatiue, it shall then be meete for him to withdrawe his mind to corporall actions of grosser sort: that as the mind by speculation, after a sort disioyneth it selfe from the bodie: so the bodily exercise may reuoke it againe into the former fellowship, and exercise of bodily action. The outwarde senses because they consist rather in a kinde of passion, their vse doth not greatly hinder the thinnesse, which we require against melancholie, except they be ouer trauelled with watching, which hath great force to drinke vp the spirites & moisture, and so to alter the bodily state into a melancholie disposition, tedious to mind and body. In their actes it is to be obserued, that they be not in anie respect irkesome, or odious. For if they be such, the heart continually where the obiect is presented, nowe growne tender thorough the internall passion, flieth at the shadow of euerie thing that carrieth the smallest shewe of discontentment: and reclaiming his spirites about him selfe, leaueth the outwarde partes destitute of conuenient measure, and by aboundance about it selfe, corrupteth them in time, for want of sufficient respiration and breathing; which no lesse ingendreth melancholie, then the former disorders afore mentioned; and as for the fearefull passion, it increaseth it directly, and keepeth that immoderate feare in vre.

Of

all sensible obiectes, the visible, except they be pleasaunt, and proportionall, giue greatest discontentment to the melancholike. If besides their horriblenesse of shape, (or without it) they represent anie significant type of tragicall calamitie, or mention that, wherewith the melancholicke apprehension faigne anie fearefull obiect: much more such spectacles are to be shunned of the melancholickes. And because darkenesse is as it were a patterne of death, it also is as much as may be to be auoyded, and all cheerefull sights, agreeable to vertue and pietie, and to be embraced, and sought after; which as the other sorte, close vp the spirites, and geueth the heart assaults of hostilitie, may allure them out againe, and set free the distressed affection, and yeelde comfort to the amazed heart. Next to visible thinges, the audible obiect most frighteth the melancholicke person, especialy besids the vnpleasantnesse, if it carieth also signification of terror: & here as pleasant pictures, and liuely colours delight the melancholicke eye, and in their measure satisfie the heart, so not onely cheerefull musicke in a generalitie, but such of that kinde as most reioyceth is to be sounded in the melancholicke eare: of which kinde for the most part is such as carieth an odde measure, and easie to be discerned, except the melancholicke haue skill in musicke, and require a deeper harmonie. That contrarilie, which is solemne, and still: as dumpes, and fancies, and sette musicke, are hurtfull in this case, and serue rather for a disordered rage, and intemperate mirth, to reclaime within mediocritie, then to allowe the spirites, to ſtirre the bloud, and to attenuate the humours, which is (if the harmony be wiſely applyed) effectuallie wrought by muſicke. For that which reaſon worketh by a more euident way, that muſicke as it were a magicall charme bringeth to paſſe in the mindes of men, which being forſeene of wiſe law giuers in times paſt, they haue made choice of certaine kindes thereof, and haue reiected the other, as hurtfull to their common wealthes; which agreement betwixt concent of muſicke, and affection of the minde, when Ariſtophenes perceaued, he therby was moued to thinke, that the mind was nothing elſe but a kind of harmonie. In the other ſenſes the obiectes onely are to be choyſed, ſweete in taſt, pleaſant in ſmell, and ſoft to be felt, that all outward things may allure, and giue courage in ſteed of that cowardly timiditie wrought by the humour. Motion doth much more, if it be vehement, and drawe to the nature of labour, and withall continuall. For that drieth the bodie exceſſiuely. And although for the preſent it be hotter through ſuch trauell: yet conſuming the ſpirite and moyſture, which are matter of this heate: in the ende it decayeth alſo, as fire without fuell, and the lampe without oyle. As theſe actions of bodie and minde being ouer vehement, and exceſſiue bereaue the humour of ſpirite, and waſte the naturall heat, which being ſpent, whatſoeuer elſe is of the body is more groſſe and earthie, & becommeth a lake of me-

lan-

lancholie: euen so if altogether these actions cease, that neither the minde nor bodie bestow themselues in good studies and exercises, then on the contrary part this worketh the same that the other excesse doth: and euen as water that standeth, and is not stirred, corrupteth, & waxeth grosse and thicke; and like as the lampe that wanteth aire goeth out, though plenty of oyle be ministred; euen so without this stirring of spirites, humours, & blood, all settle into a grosse residence of melancholie, and the whole masse of bloud easily degenerateth vnto that humour and for want of exercise the naturall fire being slakened, and the spirite thereby ingrossed, that which indued with both with iust measure, and equalitie conuenient, was before a cheerefull iuyce comfortable to all the parts, and a sweete deawe to the earthy substance, congealeth into a grossenesse farre vnmeet for that vse, and of a quite contrarie disposition.

Chap. XXXVIII.

How melancholicke persons are to order themselues in their affections.

AS in studies, exercises of the braine, sense, & voluntary motion, great moderation is to be kept of melancholy persons: euen so no lesse regarde (if not more) is to be had of them in restrayning their affectiõs, and guiding them with such wise conduct, as at no time they breake forth into outrage, and shake of the gentle and light yoake which reason imposeth. I will not now dispute whether vehement study, or disorderly perturbations is more to be taken heed of onely take you no lesse care in the one then in the other, except you finde your selfe to haue fallen into excesse, and to haue surfeted more of this, then of that excesse: If you haue so vnequally exceeded, and the effect hath preuayled with you: that kind, wherof you haue most cause to complaine, there refraine, and employ those giftes of wisedome, and vertue wherein in times past you haue bene a patterne to others: and there keepe the straightest hand, where the lists of reason are most like to be broke through. You haue had declared how the excessiue trauaile of animall actions, or such as springe from the braine, waist and spende that spirite which as it is in the world the only cheerer of all thinges, & dispenseth that life imparted of God to al other creatures, so in mans nature, is the only comfort of the terrestriall members: which spirite being consumed, or empaired, leaueth the Massy parts more heauie, grosse, and dull, and farther of remoued from all prompt, and laudable action of life: this effect as it is wrought by that kinde of disorder, in like manner, a perturbation wheron reason sitteth not, and holdeth not the raine, is of the same aptnes to disturbe the goodly order, disposed by iust proportion in our bodies: & putting the parts of that most consonāt, & pleasant harmony out of tune deliuer a note, to the great discontentment of reason, and much against the mindes will, which intendeth far other, then the

corpo-

Of Melancholie.

corporall instrument effecteth. If you will call to minde histories, you may remember how some haue died of sorrow, and othersome of ioy, and some with feare, some with ielousie, and othersome with loue: haue bin bereaued of their witts euen those most excellent in al the parts of reason, and sound vnderstanding, and therby haue made such perturbance of spirit in their braines that for credite of wisedome, and in steade of reputation: of discreite men they haue through these latter kindes of vnbridled affections, worthely caried the name of fooles, and men voide of all discreete consideration, in the whole race of their life following. This commeth to passe in some by troubling of spirite only which require nor alone due quantity, and temper, but a calme setling, and tranquillity, moued indifferently, as iust matter of perturbation shall giue occasion. In othersome by lauish waste, and predigall expence of the spirite in one passion, which dispensed with iudgement, would suffice the execution of many worthy actions besides. Hereto may furthermore adde, that as a member of the corporall body ouer vehemētly forced by straining, is in perill of luxation, & sometimes thereby becommeth altogether disioynted, and the parte looseth the freedome of flexible motion, euen so the spirite, ouerforcible strained to one vehement passion: carieth the disposition of the parte therewith, and in giuing ouer by too much yeelding to the violence of our passion, stādeth as it were crooked that way, and with an ouer reach of the raigning perturbation, being past recouery, inclineth wholly whereto it was forcibly driuen. Wherefore the perturbations are discreetely so to be ruled as alwayes there do remaine sufficient power in reasons hande to restraine. Of these some perturbations directly & immediatly increase both passion and humour, of which sorte are saddenes, and feare. Other some passing measure, not so much of theselues procure either, as they doe feeble the melancholicke bodies, as anger, and ioy, both by excessiue effusion of spirites, and suddaine alteration from the heartes contraction to such dilatation as those affections procure. In ioy if it breake forth into immoderat laughter: then doth it more feeble the melancholickes, and breath out there spirites and leaue a paine in their sides and bellies which partes are greatly trauailed in laughter. For although it should seeme meete in respect of the thinning of the humor by flowing of spirite, and blood into the outward partes from the inward center, and alteration of the passion by the contrary affection, yet the feeblenes of their bodies, and skant of spirites their humors being vnapt for plentiful supplie, respect not that consideration, but require such an expulsion of one affection by the other, that the bodie it selfe notwithstanding sustaine no detrement: otherwise the combate would be so sore, that nature not being able to beare the force of ech passion, would be dissolued by violence of that contention. So that as all matter of feare is to be abandonned, excessiue ioy is also to be eschewed as a great feebler of melancholick persons, chiefly

if

if they be women, or of tender and rare habite. If the melancholie rise of any perturbation, that especially is to be altered, & brought into a mediocrity wherof the passion take first beginning. Among them feare, and heauines are of most force, and as they are procured according to the vehemency of the cause, so the kinde of heauines and feare more or lesse encoũtereth reason, and frighteth the melancholicke heart. We both feare, and are sadde for the losse of those things which with delight and pleasure in time past we enioyed, and are tormented with despaire, and griefe when (in those thinges which we desire,) there is no hope to lay hold on. Among the sundrie sortes of subiectes to these passions, some are of necessity, and some of pleasure. Such as are of necessity either respect the natural maintenance of our bodies and liues, or honest reputation amongest men. The naturall maintenãce of life is of such force in this case that it moueth beyonde measure euen the wisest and most setled, and admitteth no moderation. If it be imbecillitie of body & voide of paine it is borne more tolerable. Reputation, mẽ of vertuous, and couragious disposition tender as their liues: wherby they are in a manner in like case and sometimes more affected with hazard thereof, then if life were in daunger. The reason is because credite and estimation toucheth the whole person of the man, and not either minde or body onely, & hath the least meanes (being oncelost) to be recouered againe, and besides the disgrace in this life, man (being immortall in soule) standeth in awe of the perpetual note of infamy which may remaine after his death. This passion is most hardlie borne of the ambitious and proude man in respect of that opinion he entertaineth of his owne worthines: & next vnto him it setleth deep in the minde enlarged with the vertue called magnanimitie, in respect his honor aunswereth not his merites. The objectes which are pleasant, if they be naturall, and not belonging to any one part, but vnto the whole nature, of which sorte is that loue which vpholdeth the propagation of kinde, and is the onely glue to couple the ioynts of this great frame of the world together: Here reason is often times failed of the passion, and (carried captiue) submitteth where it should haue preeminéce, & rule. If it be of other things which nature hath not so wedded together, the losse is borne with more tolleration, and where there is peril of want in them, despaire toucheth more lightly. In respect of their owne nature such is the condition of the thinges we desire in this world. But because the diuerse qualities of men taketh them sometimes otherwise: therfore that passion and those occasions most vrge as the partie is therwith most passionate: some one way, some an other, as nature bendeth, or education hath framed. In these cases of griefe and heauines first of all instruction out of the Scriptures of God is to be ministred, and embraced, which offering the assuraunce of farre better thinges, then the price of all wordly treasures, may swallow vp whatsoeuer calamitie this vale of miserie presseth vpon vs: next, preceptes of

morall

morall vertue and patience, with examples of constancie, and moderaton in like cases ought to moue, and consideration of that vncertaintie of pleasure in this world, which is only constant in inconstancie, and as the heauens them selues stand not still, and the nature of things receaue continual cōsuming like a streame that passeth: euen so our state is subiect vnto like mutabilitie, and with no other condition is our life deliuered vnto vs of nature, through that original disobedience, nor is to be otherwise accepted of wise men. In this case I referre the melancholick to the bookes of the Scriptures, and morall precepts of Philosophers, to the godly instructions of the diuines, and comfort of their friends. If loue not aunswered againe with like kindnesse, procure this passion, either amendes is that way to be made, or the melancholick is to be perswaded the subiect of that he liketh is not so louely, and all mention, and signification of that kind is not once to be called into minde, but whatsoeuer iustly may be alleadged to the parties disgrace is to be obiected vnto the amorous melancholicke, and other delights brought in in steed, and more highly commended, which all I leaue to the prudencie of those that attend vpon this kind of cure. And if no other perswasion will serue a vehement passion, of another sort is to be kindeled, that may withdrawe that vaine and foolish sorowe into some other extremity, as of anger, or some feare ministred by another occasion, then that which first was authour of this sadnesse. For although they both breed a dislike, yet that proceedeth of other cause, rebateth the force of it which gaue first occasion, and as one pinne is driuen out with another, so the later may expell the former: but this is to be vsed in regard of the conceit, and affection. If the body therby be altered, and the bloud thickened into melancholie, then all kind of greeuance, is to be shunned, and onely pleasaunt, and delectable things to be admitted. Thus much for the melancholicke affection, how it is to be moderated and guided: other kinds of actions, of body, are not any causes of this passion, except in such as were wont by periods to be purged of certayne melancholick bloud: which (if it faile and minister cause, or increase of this humour,) is to be diminished by opening a vaine, that may most conueniently supply that want of nature, and disburthen it of the superfluitie, as cause shall require, and force, & strength will permit. Ease and rest although it be alone of small power to ingender, yet may it be an helping cause to the passion, & increase of this humour, so that here in mediocritie is to be kept, and exercise of one sort or other neuer to be omitted, as the chiefe temper of the spirits with the humours, & quicknesse of corporall actions. For as sleepe resembleth death, and rest of the members is their kind of sleepe, & doth that in particulars which sleepe doth in the whole, so (if it excede) as ech resemble other in nature, in effect they will not be much vnlike: but as the one cooleth the bodie, and corrupteth the bloud, and extinguisheth naturall heate, whose extinction is death

it

it selfe, euen so the other in a degree hinder the present expressing of that liuely vigour, which they possesse, and disableth them afterwarde to make proofe of the facultie, wherewith they are indued. And thus haue you in these two Chapters what gouernment melancholicke persons are to obserue in their actions, and deedes that concerne maintenance of health: in the next, I will lay open vnto you of the outwarde meanes of sustentation of life what choise is to be made, and with what discretion such reliefe is to be vsed.

Chap. XXXIX.

Howe melancholick persons are to order thē selues in the rest of their diet, and what choise they are to make of ayre, meate, aud drinke, house, and apparell.

The rest of diet, consisteth in the right vse of outward sustentation of life, which is either taken inward, or is outwardly vsed only. The inward and such as is to be receaued into our bodies: is either aire, or sustenance. The ayre meet for melancholicke folke, ought to be thinne, pure and subtile, open, and patent to all winds: in respect of their témper, especially to the South, and Southeast, except some other imbecillity of their bodies dissuade therefrom, and in the contrarie part, marrish, mistie, and foggie ayre is to be eschued as an increase of both humour, and passion. Sustenaunce is either meate or drinke. Their meates ought not onely to be chosen such as of their owne nature do ingender to pure and thinne iuyce, but if the nature of the nourishment be otherwise, the preparation ought to giue it a correction of that fault, and generallie they should be liquide, and in forme of brothes, that both by the moyst qualitie thereof, the drinesse of the humour, and their bodies might be refourmed, and that the passage & concoction might also be more easie, and speedy in all their partes. Nourishmentes of their owne nature among meats, wholsome and meet for melancholicke folke, and of vegetable things, are parsnep, carret, and skerret roots. And sallet herbs, lettice, mallowes, and endiue mixed with a quantitie of rocket, and taragon, are not to be refused, no more is aretch, sorell and purslane with the late twaine aboue mentioned, or with persley, charuell and fenell, with litle vineger, plenty of oyle and suger. Of sorts of bread, cheat bread, is meetest for them, and if they be charged with store of bloud, and the vaines full, some oates, barley, or millet flower mingled with the wheat meele, shall abate the aboundant nourishment of the wheat. Of frutes, such as are moyst, soft, and sweet are meetest for them, as the iuyce, damsing, cherrie, figges, grapes, and abricots: neither are newe walnuts, and greene almonds hurtfull in this case. Capers washed from the salt and vineger, and eaten with suger and oyle are meeter for them then oliues. Of flesh, the young is fittest for their diet, and the younger the better, in respect of their colde and drie bodies, and grosse humours, which require plentifull

OF MELANCHOLIE.

tifull moystening and warming, which is supplyed by the tender age of those things whereof we feede: being fuller of vitall heate, and naturall moysture, then the older of the same kind. Neither is it requisite that they be young onely, but also well liking, and of the same kinde the tame, and domesticall is meete for correction of their melancholicke state, then the wilde. Againe of flesh, the foule is to be preferred for their vse before the beast, and that foule rather which vseth much the feete, and lesse the wing. Of foule these are of especiall choyce for melancholicke persons, the partridge, the godwit, the yong pigeon, the pullet, the feasant, & the yong turky, among these the goose wing hath his place, not to be refused if the melancholicke haue appetite thereto. And generally of foule the carued is better, then the other. Of beastes the gelded haue preferment aboue their felowes of that kind: among them pigge is meet for melancholy, farced with sage and such like art of cookerie, to dry vp part of his superfluous humiditie: veale, especially of a cowe calfe, yong wether mutton, kidde, & rabbet are of the best kind of diet among the beasts for melancholick persons. Of the pattes of flesh: the brawnes and muscles are the best, and next to them the tong is of second choyce. Of liuers, the pigges liuer among beasts is the best, & the stones of cockerells yeeld commendable nourishment. Of flesh these aboue mentioned are most agreable with the diet cure of melancholie, & such parts of thẽ as I haue declared: the other either breeding

R iij

a grosse, or slimie nourishment hard of digestion and slowe of passage. Generally fish is not so wholsome as flesh for this vse, because they be not so well stored with naturall heate and moysture, except the imbecillitie of the melancholick stomach be such as wil not beare the strégth of flesh, then is the fish to be boyled with wine, and to be eaten out of some wholesome broth, or with good store of sweet butter, and sauoured with pepper. If the partie desire fish, these following are principall among them. And first generally such as are of a middle bignesse, not too fat, nor leane, white, and brittle of substance, & haunt the swiftest and purest waters, are most commendable: for such breed subtilest nourishment, and least fraight with excrements. Of salt water fish that beare shells, the oyster is only for this diet, of those that are defended with a crust, the shrimp, and crayfish go before the rest. Of other kind of seafish, such as haunt the rockes are excellent food for melancholicke persons, corrected and vsed as I haue before shewed: as the gilthead, the whiting, the sea pearch &c. Of other sort the mullet, the lucie, the haddocke, the sole, place, but, gurnard and rotchet are to be admitted into this diet. Of fresh water fish, those of the riuer are to be preferred: & the rest scarse to be touched, except they receaue correction from the kitchin. Of riuer fish these are of the wholsomest kinde: pearch, pike, gougeon, & trout. Thus of the substance of creatures you haue what I iudge meetest for you in this case. Of the other sort, nothing is to be refused but

cow-

OF MELANCHOLIE.

cowmilke, all other sorts carrying a thinner, and more liquid substance, and importing no perill of obstruction, nor windinesse: especiallly taken with suger and a litle salt, & two or three houres before any other sustenance. As cow milk is the grossest and thickest, so mares milke (except that of camels) is the thinnest, next of asse, goats milke is most moderate, and ewes milke thicker then it. Of the partes of milke, whay drunke with suger is wholesome for melancholicke folke, neither is fresh and new butter to be refused, cheese made altogether of cowe milke is vnwholsome, mixed with goats, or asses milk, maketh it not so apt to breed obstructions. Eggs are good, and wholesome sustenance for melancholicke bodies, rosted rather then sod or potched, and reare dressed somwhat the yelk thicker then to be supped. Of egges, hens, feasaunts, and turkies lay the wholesomest egges, and are only for the melancholickes dish. Thus much concerning the meates fit for their diet. Their dressing ought to be such as may maintaine their naturall iuyce as much as may be, with remouing of all rawnesse. Their sawces would be the iuyce of an orange or lymon, well qualified with suger and sweet butter, especially if vineger or veriuyce be part in sauce, more in vineger, & lesse in veriuyce. Their drinke would be of barlie mault brued with raine water, or spring water which is much drawn of, next to these riuer water may take the third place of commendation. It would be of a midle strength, & not too stale: beare rather thē ale, becausē the hops do great-

R iiij

ly respect their liuer and splene, & scoureth the stomach, and maketh purer, and readier way for distribution of their nourishment. It shall be very good for them to drinke at meales a draught of wine of good strength: claret rather then white, and of any kind well refined, and full of wine. If they drinke their wine with suger, it giueth greater cheering to them, maketh it to passe more easily, and mitigateth their melancholicke sowrenesse. Drinke betwixt meales, or after meate is to be auoyded, except great cause vrge. Hitherto their sustenance, of what kinde it ought to be of, and among such varietie of food, and so many good blessinges of God that way, what choyce is to be made: as for their order of eating, and drinking, and measure of both, as liquid meates and brothes are most conuenient for them, so I take it, they may drinke largely, (except some accident of the stomach dissuade) By reason their digestion is slowe, my aduise is, they eate litle, and often: litle because their strength beareth not much, nor such mediocrity as other men: often, because their spirites are fewe, and neede repayring: besides the colde, sower, and setling humour of melancholie is to be refreshed as much as may be, with fresh and pure nourishment, and to be tempered, and mitigated with that sweet and gentle mixture. The outward maintenance of life, and sustentation of our fraile bodies consist in house or habitatiō, & apparell, which both must carie these properties to be cleane and nete, and in all respects as much as may be satisfying the minde of the melancho-

OF MELANCHOLIE.

lancholicke. For although meates and drinkes, and ayre, either vnwholesome, or vnpleasaunt beare great sway in disposing the humour, yet because they haue not such power to affect the minde and senses as these other haue, in respect of the passion, and melancholike affection, they worke not so present annoyaunce. The house except it be cheerefull and lightsome, trimme and neate, seemeth vnto the melancholicke a prison or dungeon, rather then a place of assured repose and rest. And the apparell except it be light, cleane, fitte, and well sitting, maketh shewe of deformitie, to the melancholicke, and being euer in his eye, is a representation of his present calamitie, verie tedious vnto him, or if it be not so in his conceit, being nowe farre altered: yet agreeing with the humour, it may be meanes of increase thereof, and augmenting the fancie. The situation of his house, or at the least of his chamber, and place where he is most conuersant, would be such as might let in such kinde of ayre as I haue before declared, & seated neither too lowe in anie bottome, nor vpon hill too high, except the melancholie be out of measure, sadde and sullen, then an high, loftie, and troubled ayre, and such seate of house will not be amisse. If the melancholicke be of abilitie, the house would not want ornament of picture, of gay and fresh colours, in such matter as shall be most pleasaunt, and delightfull, and of all ornamentes of house, and home, a pleasaunt gardin and hortyeard: with a liuelie springe, is aboue all domesticall delight, & meetest for the melancholy heart and brayne. His apparell would be decent and comely, and as the purse will giue leaue somewhat for the time sumptious, as also the whole houshold furniture belonging vnto him. Of colour, light, or chaungeable, except the place, & grauity of the melancholy person refuseth colours, and here no kinde of seemely ornament would be omitted which might entice the senses to delight, and allure the inclosed spirites to solace theselues the outward parts of their bodies: here brouches, chaines, & ringes may haue good vse with such like ornament of iewell as agreeth with the hability and calling of the melancholicke: and those not onely curious, and pretious by arte, but especially garnished with precious stones that are said to haue vertue against vaine feares and basenes of courage. Of which sorte are these following: the Carbuncle for vertue the chiefe of stones: The Calcedonye of power to put awaye feare and heauines of hearte, a cleerer of the Spirites, and chaser away of fantasticall melancholy visions. The ruby auayleable against fearfull dreames. The Iacint a great cheerer of the heart, and procurer of fauour. The Turcoyse, a comforter of the Spirites. The Chrysophars of like vertue. The Corneole a mitigater of anger and meete for molancholickes of the furious sorte. Stones of baser sorte and yet of singuler vertue, are the Chalydony, or swallow stone, found in the mawes of young swallowes, against madnes: and the Alectorian or Cockes stone, of a watery colour, found in the mawe of a Cocke or Capon after he be nine yeares olde, aboue all commended for giuing strength and courage, and wherewith (as it is reported) the famous Milo Crotonien alway stoode inuincible. Thus haue you the whole order of the melācholie diet. I doe not remember any thing particular, and peculiar vnto them necessary, more thē hath bene hitherto declared, wherefore in the next chapter I will also lay open what phisicke helpe is requisite in this case, and so recommend the successe and fruite of my labour to the blessing of God vpon you, and such as are partakers of like affliction. As for the furious melancholy, I leaue it to be cured as deseafe and sicknes, and will not meddle therewith in this place, being impertinent to my purpose, which respecteth onely your estate, and such like condition of others.

Chap. XL.

The cure by medicine, meete for melancholie persons.

BEfore I enter to treate of the cure by medicine one word of admonition touching the vse of the medicines and meanes shall be first necessary both for your sake, & others who may hereafter haue vse of this my counsell: my meaning is not to make you a phisicien, or to giue warrant by this my labour to any rashly, & without direction of the learned phisicien, to aduenture practise vpon this aduise, as the common sorte is to venterous to attempt what they read of medicine deliuered in their vulgar toung, but that seing the manifold good meanes which god in his great prouidence, and mercy hath ordained for the releefe, you may take courage in the consideratiō of his goodnes herein, and receiue refreshing by the view of his aide though it be a farre of, which the discreete application of the wise phisiciā (who is made of God for the health of men) shall bringe nigh vnto you, and ioyning with this strength of melancholy, chase it farre from you, and render vnto you the former good disposition of your body, and desired tranquillitie of your minde. For medicine is like a toole & instrument of the sharpest edge, which not wisely guided, nor handled with that cunning which thereto appertaineth, may bringe present perill in steade of health, and where it should be a succour, and maintenance of life, for want of arte, may worke a contrary effect, daungerous, and deadly. To the right applying of medicine, besides the particular considerations belonging properly to the arte of phisicke wherein exercise maketh the phisician prompt and expert, sharpe of iudgement, and circūspect in the cure, you your selfe know what furniture of philosophie is necessary, euen the whole course of arts, and knowledge of nature, but onely to prepare, and to giue hability, of conceiuing, and learning the rules of preseruing and restoring the health of mans body, which we call phisicke: so that as Galen sayeth in a booke of that title, a phisician ought

ought to be a philosopher, the best philosopher maketh the best phisician, neither ought any to be admitted to touch so holy thinges, that hath not passed the whole discipline of liberall sciences, and washed himselfe pure and cleane in the waters of wisedome, and vnderstanding. The abuse at this day is great, and commō, defrauding the simple sorte in their substance and hurting of their bodies vnder the pretence of experiéce, of secretes and hid misteries of remedies, which these masked theeues, & murtherers alleage for color of their lewdnes. That (as I am perswaded) there are not so many honest and painefull men of any one trade in the lande, as their be lewde cousoning varletts, that to auoide the trauaile of honest labour, feede vpon the simplicitie of the people, and make the pretence of phisicke the cloake of their idlenes. Othersome there be of a curiositie not knowing what they doe bould to attempt out of an english booke the practise of any recite, and will not sticke to encounter the iudgement of the wisest and best practised phisician. These are vnthankefull, and presumpteous. Vnthankefull in that they acknowledge not from whome they haue receaued these wholesome meanes: presumpteous, in hazarding the health of an other, and aduenturing their owne credit vpon the receite of a medicine with perill of life where it is bestowed, which of it selfe is but an instrument onely, and worketh good or hurte, as it is applied and guided: to the application whereof the long studies the knowledge of so many partes of philosophie and learning, the peregrinations, and conferences of learned men make proofe, and giue sufficient testimony both what is requisite, and how farre of they be from modestie and honesty that being vnfurnished altogether, of euery parte of these necessary helpes, dare attempt the application of medicine whose nature they know not and of what dispositiō the body or part is wherto it is to be applied, they are vtterly ignoraunt. But one will say they doe sometimes good: they doe so, but oftentimes hurte, and more hurt thē presently appeareth, and with that good they in one respect doe, in diuerse besides they leaue the body crased, and make it afterward subiect to greater infirmitie: there cure being imperfect, accidentall, vncertaine, void of rule and reason. wherefore although you haue for your part passed your course in philosophy & good learning and are not altogether ignoraunt of the precepts of phisicians whereby this warning might seeme lesse to appertaine vnto you, yet cōsidering your present infirmity, and vpon what graines & moments, and points of time this practise standeth: I counsell you & all other except the directiō of diet that hath binbefore declared, & vse of those familiar things w̄ euery one daily putts in practise, without the aduise of the phisician, (whose present eye may behold euery necessity,) you vtterly abstaine, and take my labour herein as a poynting of the finger to that which I iudge meet for you being in a place far distant, & wher necessity may cōpell you to vse what meanes of counsell you cā get: & not such as you woulds

and

and vpon the view of these manifold meanes of bodely health: consider how much more the Lords prouidēce is ready at all neede, to cōfort our soules, in so much as the one is far more excellent then the other. Thus hauing giuen this warning I proceed to deliuer the naturall helps and ordinarie remedies we doe vse in this case wherein your bodely health now standeth. Hetherto you vnderstād what outward causes are to be remoued, and what to be brought in stead of them, contrary in operation, and breeders of a better tempered humour. The next consideration (according to the method of curing) is to be had of such inward cause as resteth in the body, and hath bene the effect of the outward annoyance: that is here the melancholick humour, and complexion of the bodie now degenerated thereby. The humour requireth euacuation, and emptying: and because your body is not only melancholicke vnder the ribbes but the whole masse of your blood is chaunged therewith: it shall be first necessarye to open a vaine: that both thereby you may be disburthened in parte of that heauy load, and nature hauing lesse of that kinde to deale withall, may alter the remnant into a more milde and pleasant iuice: thinne it in substance, and temper it with naturall heate and moisture: in quality. Before any vaine be opened a clister is first to be receaued that may clense the entrailes and diminish some part of the humour seated in those parts, it wold be made of marshmallowes, holyhockes, pelletory of the wale, mercurie, beetes, aretch, violet leaues, polipody, borrage, bugloſſe, chammomile, hoppes, dill, and melilote, aniſe ſeeds, and fennell, decoƈted in ale or beere: and the decoƈtion being made, an ounce of Confeƈtio hamech with a drame of Hiera pichra added thereto. Hony wherein roſemarye flowers haue bene ſteeped, and oyle of dill of ech an ownce and a halfe, this or ſuch like according to the diſcretion of the learned phiſiciā. The morning following the vaines are to be emptied the neceſſity of the paſſiō compared with the force and ſtrength which moderateth all kinde of euacuatiō, though the deſeaſe require large emptying. And becauſe melandcholy blood is thicke and groſſe, & therfore eaſily flow:th not though the vaine be opened, it ſhall helpe the bleeding to exerciſe your body a while before with ſuch moderation that it be equally warmed, and the ſpirite, and blood ſtirred vp. The Orifice would be ſomewhat large that no lett be to the iſſue, & the groſſenes of the blood may haue the free paſſage: yet ſo that it be no larger then is requiſite, for waſting of ſpirits wher of melācholy perſons haue no ſtore to ſpare. In the body the middle vaine of the left arme is fitteſt to be opened, which, reſpecƈteth, both head, liuer, and ſplene: that betwixt the little finger and the next is of ſmall vſe. In ſuch as haue the adduſt melancholy ſeated in their brains, the head vaine is more direƈt for reuulſion, and thoſe about the head it ſelfe for euacuating and deriuing. The tokens of ſeating there only, are with altered fancie and imagination, the bodie elſe carying no melan-

cholicke

Of Melancholie.

cholicke signes, no fower belching after meate, nor heate with windinesse, which all rise of the melancholy humour stopping the mesaraicke vaines, and so procuring that vnnaturall & suffocating heate, which many melancholick persons complaine of. The quantitie which I would haue you spare, let it be no lesse then nine or ten ownces, except the present action of opening minister other consideration. Nowe because you haue had in times past the benefite of bleeding hemorhods, which now a long time are stopped at such seasons as they were wont to open, or now when they giue any signe of fulnesse, swelling or paine, they would also be opened by applying a redde onion to the place, or annointing it with the iuyce of garlicke, or with bulles gall, or rubbing it with a figge leafe, or with horsleeches well purged, and prepared, and so applied the easiest way: by opening the inwarde vaines of the ankle, & such like remedies as may prouoke the bloud his vsuall way, and bring nature in minde of her wonted discharge of that humour, which being stopped breedeth (as Hipocrates saith, and experience maketh proofe) frensies, melancholies, pleurisies, hard milts, & dropsies: and contrarily opened, & flowing moderatly, deliuereth from them all. If this melancholy falleth vnto maidens, or women, & their ordinarie course faile them, the vaines of the hammes or ancles are to be cut, and drinkes of opening rootes, fenell, persly, butchers brome, madder, and such like, with germander, goolds, herbe grace, mugwort and nep are to be much

S

vsed, with sittinges and bathinges in mallowes, chammomile and nep, peniroyall, bay leaues, fetherfew (and such like), which haue vertue in that case) decocted in water, wherein so much honie hath bene dissolued, as will giue it a tast of sweetnesse: if greater force be required then a dramme of the troches of myrre in the former decoctiō are most forcible, the opening of vaine before mentioned would be procured at the accustomed time, at the full mone in the elder sort, and the chaunge in the yonger. The thicker the bloud is, the more the melancholick may spare, and the thinner, the lesse. Thus much I iudge necessarie for one kind of euacuation, which although it letteth out good bloud withall (as in all bleeding) yet here lyeth the benefit, that nature is partly disburthened, and so more easilie gouerneth the rest, and by vertue of her natural heate, and spirit, correcteth with smaller helpe that which therin is farther to be reformed, the spirites haue free libertie, and great scope is giuen to the harts dilating, the action peculiar to a cheerfull disposition. The other kinde of euacation is by purging: which leaueth the bloud entrie, only it cleanseth the bodie of that grosse and thicke settelinge, and is more peculiar, and directly singleth out the melancholie from the other humours: and because this humour is thicke, and hardly moueth, and the passages, & veines of the body closer then whereby it may easily passe, (according to Hipocrates rule) both bodie and humour are to receaue a preparation, and the parts of the body to be loosened,

and

and enlarged, & the humor made more flowing and thinne, both which may be brought to passe with one meanes at once: by choyce of such natures as haue vertue of attenuating, opening, & cleansing: and because the cure is not onely intended against the melanchólicke humour, and that complexion of body, but also against the fancy, and affection, which we call in phisicke symptomes, alwayes choice would be made of such as carrie with them proprietie to strengthē the altered braine, and to cheere the comfortlesse hart: or if that cannot be found in one simple, it is to be supplied by mixture. Their temper would be moderate in heat, except the naturall temper of the body, time of yeare, sex &c. (and such like considerations) perswade on either side any declination. The simples meete for this preparation of body, & humour are these which follow: borrage, buglosse, endiue, fumitory, hops, betony, the sorts of maidē haire, ceterach, harts tong, polypody, doddar of thime, agrimony, cich pease, ash barks, caper barks, tamarisk, to which would be added opening roots, fenell, persley, smallage, butchers broome, alparagus, and such like. Of these simples decoctions shold be made, and mixed with syrops of like vertue, as with syrope of borrage, of apples, simple, or compound, as that of King Sabor, syrope of fumitory, syrope of violets, of ceterach, syrope of epithymus or doddar of thime: all openers of splene and liuer, cleansers of the bloud, & great preparers to the purging both of bodie, and humour: the vse of them would be much, & often fasting that they may haue their ful force. Moreouer to this vse a kind of beare, brued with the simples before mentioned, and some small relish of cloues and cynamon giuen vnto it: & so vsed as ordinary drinke would be very wholsome for melancholick persons: and now and then if the stomach be raw & rheumatick, a draught of hippocras, or some aromaticall wine giueth great comfort, increaseth the spirits, and maketh the bloud thinne. But here heede must be giuen that it be not too strong of spice, least through too much heate, by euaporatinge the thinne part, the rest of the bloud remaine more thicke, and harder to be purged. Besides these inwarde preparations, and opening and thinning potions, the liuer, and the splene, and the partes vnder the ribs would be suppled with conuenient fomentations and oyntmentes, to soften to open, & to loosen those parts where the purging medicin hath most to do: this may be done with fomentations made of mallowes, chammomile, melilot, figges, lineseede, fetherfew, rewe, and rose leaues, red and damaske, and the part being a while supplied therwith, some mollsying and warming ointment is to be rubbed & chafed in gently, with a soft hand: as that which is called cōmonly resumptiuū, the oyntment of briony, the ointment of swines bread called cyclamen, vpon which if need be a plaister of like effect may haue very good vse, as diachylum magnum, the emplaister of melilote for the splene: ceroneum, diamelilotum of Andramachus &c. to these preparatiōs, & disposings of body, & humour

Of Melancholie. 275

mor to the purging. If it seme good vnto the phisitiās, & for varietie, baths would be vsed of mollifying & moderatly warming simples, as of mallowes, marsh mallowes, holihock, chammomile, melilot, peniroyall, lineseed, roses, &c. In which decoction lukewarme, the body is to be kept half an houre at a time (or as present occasion shall direct) fasting, & in the while the partes vnder the short ribbes suppled & exercised with a soft hand, anointed with oyle of capers: oile of bitter alomonds, & a fewe drops of petroleum mixed therwith. After the body hath bin thus prepared & the humour somwhat more loose, & easie to moue: purgation is next to be attēpted: by stoole rather then by vomit, except the party be verie apt therunto, and the melancholy be chiefly seated therabout. The simples proper to purge melancholy are these following: Sena, polypodie, blacke hellebore, and white, the azure stone, and more gentle then it, the Armenian stone, all which diligently prepared and corrected, & ministred in quantity meet for the patients strēgth enter combat with this humor, & with such force chaseth it out of the body, that it followeth it euen into the stoole. The compounds are diasena confectio hamech: hieralogadion: pils of fumitory, Inde of the azure, and Armenian stone, in which the simples before mentioned receaue their correction, & due preseruation, farre more safe to be vsed then the simple alone, all which purgers are to be receiued & mingled with some moysting decoction, as of barley, with borrage, buglosse, violet leaues, & syrope of violetets, bor-

S iij

rage, buglosse &c. if they be electuaries, or powders, & if they be pils, a thin broth, drunke inmediatly after them, that both the liquid substance may giue a speedy conueyance, & the dry humor soked with that forme of medicine, may more gently yeeld, & giue place to the purge. Whē the medicine is felt now to haue passed the stomach which is perceaued that it yeeldeth no medicinable taft to the mouth, by belching or breath, then some broth may be také, made of such kind of flesh & herbs as haue bene before mentioned, and so (till the working cease) the whole action of the medicine to be endured. Thus much for purging by stoole: if vomit be thought more necessarie, (as I iudge it very necessarie in you) whatsoeuer emptieth the stomach by prouoking nature that way (except the matter be very hard to moue, & deep setled) shall suffise for that sort of euacuation. Vomit is very necessary when the stomach is moist & watery, and maketh shewe therof by much spitting, whē the patient is troubled with soure belching, and when the meate is perceaued (in mouing of the body) to be loose, & iogge in the stomach: then I say all other circūstāces cōcurring together, vomit is to be vsed: first of the gentle sort: of which kinde are radish roots, & seeds, pompeon root, netle seed, astrabacka root or leafe &c. if the cause & strength of the melancholick require a greater force of medicine, Stibium, & white hellebore are singular in this case: which both would be ministred in fat broth: the substance of Stibium, & the infusion of neesing powder or white helleborus: being in
substance

substance most daungerous. This kind of hellebore more helpeth the fancy, and correcteth the braine, and the other more dealeth with the humour, & both discretly vsed performe a most wholsome euacuation. If the melancholicke do labour much in vomiting, minister drinke or thin broth, so shall the vomit be with more ease discharged. All perturbation of the bodie being ended, & the medicine hauing wrought the desired effect, the face is to be refreshed with some mixture of rosewater, and vineger, and rose water is to be smelled vnto, the mouth to be washed and some conserue of red roses, with a quarter so much of quince preserued, and one drop of oyle of cloues, or cynamon, would be receaued to strengthen the stomach againe, to settle it quiet, & if any quality of the medicine remaine to correct & alter it, what soeuer therby the stomach should feele of discontentment. This emptying of stoole & vomit, is so often to be repeated, & by such distace of time, as need requireth: the strength of the melancholick will beare, and the humor admitteth of preparation: especially the spring & fall craue this emptying at large.

Chap. XLI.

The maner of strengthning melancholick persons after purging: with correction of some of their accidents.

Betwixt the spaces of purging regard is alwayes to be had of strengthening the stomach liuer, and splene, with some ointment and fomentatiō outwardly, of a moderate astrictiue vertue, and some inward medicine compounded of such simples as are accompted familiar, and simpatheticall to those partes: as of inward thinges, to the stomach mintes, betony wormewood, suger roses, mastites, galaga, mace, cloues, cinnamon, amber ginger. &c, of which, potions, powders, and electuaries would be made, and vsed for the stomach. Of the same matter fomentations would also be made, especially of Cammomill, roses, wormewood, and agrimony. Of compoundes conserue of wormewood, of sage flowers, of Enula campana, of mintes are singuler comforters of the stomach and bowels: the same vertue haue greene walenuts preserued, embliske, myrobolans, and greene ginger: lozēges of Aromaticum rosatum, Dianisi. The ointementes are to be made of red roses, corrall, masticke, mintes, cloues, cinnamon, gumme, aloes, with oyle of wormewood, masticke, quinces. &c, and here the emplaister of a crust of bread, described of montagnana greatly strengtheneth the stomake, as also the stomach plaister of mesue. For the liuer these are meetest strengtheners: liuerwoorte, maiden heare, agrimony, fumitory hoppes, asparagus, wormewood, horehound, germander, saunders, yuorie roses, raysinges, runcus odoratus, Calamus aromaticus. &c, of which stuffe potions, powders, electuaries are to be receiued inwardly, and fomentations, oyles, ointments, and plaisters to be applied outwardly. Of compoundes conserue of fumitory conserue of wormewood, conserue of maiden heare, Dialacca, Diacurcuma, Diaçostum, open obstructions, and leaue a strengthening vertue in the part: of the splene, hoppes,

dod-

doddar, ceteracoke, heath, caper barkes, tamariske, acorus, gumme lacca, centaurie be peculiar comforters. Of inward compoundes: diacosthum: diacalamentum, diacappairis, conserue of ceterach Of outward meanes, oyle of capers, oyle of spike, and oyle of lillies compounded with maslich, cloues, cinnamon, saffrone, costus, and Calamus aromaticus are openers and comforters of the splene: and of oyntmentes, martiatum magnum: of plaisters, Diaphenicon, &c. These wholesome medicines after the purges haue satisfied the phisicians intention, would be vsed and much applied both in respect of the parties disposition through the melancholicke humor, and also by reason these doe sustaine the greatest force of purgations, and preparations afore said: and whose natures are easily dissolued, and alwayes require a strengthening simple mixt with the rest: though they be of contrary operation. In the meane while of this preparation, and purging: both in respect of the fancy, of the brayne, and affection of the hearte, and the complexion of both, put out of frame by the humour, these two are chiefely to be respected, with cordialls, and medicines appropriate. Cordiall, simples are these: borrage, buglosse, the iuice of pippins and parmaines, balme, Carduus benedictus, scabions, basill seede, vincois horad, beasar stone, yuorie, pearle saphyre, iacint, corall, amber, limon, and citron pile, cinnamon cloues, wine, suffran, angellica, marygooldes, with a number of like nature, the great prouidence of God being such that this noble part of the hearte hath moe helpes and comforts peculiar thereunto, then any parte of our body besides. The compoundes vsuall are these: conserue of borrage, and buglosse flowers, of orāge flowers, of gillyflowers, and carnations, diamagaritō calidum, the electuary of pretious stones, letificans Galeni mithridate dianthos, &c. Of the decoction of which hearbs afore mentioned, epithemes may be made, and quilts of the powder of them, besprinckled with malmsey & vineger. Which forme of outward medicine made of simples agreeable to the stomach is good thereto also to be applied: whose mouth doth greatly agree with the hearte, and easily driueth into passion. As the hearts affection is to be corrected, by amending the instrumēt: so the braines conceite requireth no lesse regard: for which these medicines, following are yeelded to our cōfort: sage, betony, sweet mariorume, rosemary, chāmomil, mirtle, rue, peony, spite, storax, benoyne cloues muske, amber greece. Of compoundes: cōserue of rosemary flowers, of acorns of betony, of stechas, sage, peony, and primerose Dambra, Diamoschum dulce, and amarum. Neither is the braine and heart only cheered, & cōforted by the inward receiuing of these simples only, but whatsoeuer of them is of pleasant and fragraunt smell, that agreeth with ech, & giueth recreation and increase to the spirits of both. So that sweete smels are both in respect of hearte and braine most comfortable to the melancholicks. Thus the melācholick body, dieted, prepared, purged, & strengthened, what is there more

to

Of Melancholie.

to be done of naturall meanes: only this: After all this course taken, and diligently obserued so long as it shall seeme expediét and necessary to the learned phisiciā for the health of this melācholick patient, (among whome I accompt you the subiect of this my coūsell) nature must haue a time and respit giuen, to try her owne strégth, according to the counsell of Ruphus, and not to be tiered with medicine, the diet notwithstāding being kept diligently which hath bin prescribed and all kinde of honest exercise, and recreation practised & procured. If the melācholy be adust, (which it is not in you) then breedeth it a kinde of fury, and madnes, and requireth a cooling: & perticular consideration: whereof (because it is very rare in respect of the other kinde, & entereth into the rancke of euident desease) I minde not here to discourse being only willing thus far to satisfie your desire, wherein your case (& such as are in like códitió with you,) require it. If any accidentes befall you through this infirmity, of hardnes of body you may yse the clifter before mentioned without the purging medicines, with three ownces of oyle, and as much of hony: or you may take an handefull of mallowes, holy-lock, violet leaues, beete, and fetherfew, annise seedes, or fennell seedes halfe an ounce beaten with an handfull of course whete branne tied in a linné cloth & boyled in thinne whay: to a pint of which being strained, adde oyle, and honie, with halfe a spoonefull of salt: and receiue it for a clister: or drinke fasting a spoonefull or twayne of sweete sallet oyle in a draught of whay, or eate a quarter of an ownce of conserue of damaske roses, with xxx. graines of the purest salt peter, and drinke it: and especially let your broathes alwayes haue some soluble heurbes, that may giue you that benefite, as mallowes, violettes, mercurie, aretch, beetes and such like. If your sleepe fayle you through vehemency of cogitation, and feare: let your hands and feete be washed with the decoction of dill, chammomill, lettice, poppie mallowes, and willowe leaues: and annointe them with oyle of poppie seedes made by expression: or take a dramme of Mithridate, fiue graines of Opium three of saffron, with a spoonefull of malmesey, and a graine or two of Camphire: put all into a limon pill emptied of the iuice, and smell to it often about your ordinary hower of sleep: which meanes if they bring not the desired effect, swallow twenty graines of the piles of Cynoglosse, or take halfe a dramme of Philomum going to bed for other some other wholesome opiats medicine well corrected. If your body be much troubled with winde (as it is for the most part a companion of this kinde of melancholy:) yee must vse a fomentation to your stomach bellie and partes about the short ribbes with oyle and malmesey wherein rue, fennell, cumine, and anise seedes, and hearbs haue bene boyled, and inwardly you are to take fasting Deatrion piptrion, diaciminu, or diagalanga the quantitie of a nutmegge at a time: and now and then cerecloath of gummes, with oyle of mints, and rue, worne vpon those partes, shall be of great force to waſt the winde, to warme them, and to giue them ſtrength. Thus my friende *M.* haue you my whole counſell, what I iudge meete for you in this caſe, my philoſophicall diſcourſes to paſſe your time with, who hath alwayes delighted in philoſophie: my conſolation in reſpect of that Chriſtian duety which I owe you, wherein if I haue ſo buſied my ſelfe, that my care that waye hath exceeded my power,& hability,ſo eſteeme it, and ſo meaſure that diſcharge. My phiſicke, cure: of diet, of preparation of your body, of euacuation, of ſtrengthening, of correcting, and cutting of certaine troubleſome accidẽts that fall to this humour, it is not ſo copious, and abſolute as peraduenture may fitte your eſtate, & leaue no queſtion of doubt, but (if I miſtake not the caſe very much) for ſubſtance and grounde of the cure you ſhall not neede to make farther inquirie Although I remember your trauaile in philoſophie, and ſtudie of phiſick, to which both you haue had a naturall diſpoſition, and take pleaſure in reading our writinges of precept & rule take aduiſe of ſome learned, and vertuous phiſician about you, and aduenture not vpon any part of euacuation without his direction: Otherwiſe you haue this as a touchſtone to proue the skill of ſuch lewde people as at this day are impudently bold with the hurte of others, to deceiue boaſting,& lying, and couering the pouertie of their vnderſtanding, with gorgeous wordes, and rich pompe of phraſe: otherwiſe being as empty of knowledge as they be quite void of all vertue and honeſty. I ſay let it be a rule to square and try them by: and if such knowledge (whereof here you may haue the taft) be neceſſary in an infirmity of no perill of life (though it make it tedious, and irkeſome) what aduiſement and care is to be had whome to call for, & what phiſician to make choice of in deſeaſes full of daunger, ſharp, and ſwift, and whoſe cure (if art be not in all pointes perfourmed) is not without leauing ſuch ſcar, that no rebating, no deterſiue medicine is able to pare & wipe away the blemiſh: not an eye ſore, but a maime, and fixed imbecillitie in ſtomach, in braine, in hart, or liuer, nor that by natures error, or by an ordinarie breach of diet which are more gentle, but through an outward violence and force, againſt which nature hath no skill to helpe it ſelfe, nor power to reſiſt. As I giue you this warning to beware, ſo whoſoeuer ſhall reape any fruit of my labour taken in hand for your ſake, let them alſo take this admonition from me, rather then to attend with their own hurt, & expence, the inſtruction & diſcipline which experience bringeth. Thus my good *M*. with this caueat, I commend the bleſſing & ſucceſſe of my labour to the Almighty, who reſtore you if it be his will ſound in bodie, cheerfull in mind, and aſſured in faith of his ſweete mercie and fauour.

FINIS.

Faults escaped in the printing, wherein the first number signifieth the page, the 2. the line.

For materiall, naturall. 4. 2. for any an. 6. 30. for was, were 8. 10. for aſſimulate, aſſimilate. 10. 11. for in of. 12. 33. for enioyeth, enioy. 17. 19. for and, an. 20 27. for fitteth, ſitteth therewith. 21. 8. for our, other 21. 27. for then the. 21. 39. for to, of. 20. 11. for act, art. 20. 13. by an accidentall, put out by. 24. 23. for recouery, may. 26. 1. ot and from their, or from. 27. 18. for haue the pooles, haunt the. 29. 7. for miſlie, miſty. 30. 21. for in that, that. 39 4. for being, beginning. 51. 9. If you wil diſcend &c. 54. 19 ſhould follow decayeth. l. 13. for then, the. 57. 27. put out it. 68. 11. for wherof thereof. 74. 13. for depending, depēd 77. 4. for lightly, rightly. 79. 13. for is, it. 85. 5. ſo is ouermatched, and is ouermatched. 86. 5. put out by 103. 15. be offered. 104. 21. impoſſible, as I take it. 118. 18. put out by 131. 23. ouercharged. 141. 19. this greedineſſe. 131. 3. proneneſſe of nature. 134. 10. benummet. 139, 5 diſtractiō 140 1. our moſt deare. 140. 13. one and the other. 141. 8. cords. 157. 27. both laughing. 161. 15. put out the firſt &. 163. 11. ovvne heat. 165. 19. the body. 165. 20. either in doing. 168. 4. exſpiration. 169. 30. neere neighbourhood, 175 17. vehement reuenge of him ſelf for the offence. 167. 8. barbarous. 193. 14. ſucceſſe. 222 17. put out of. 124. 29 put out the. 158. vlt. for diſtruction, diſtraction. 140. 1. put out hinder. 144. vlt. put out large 160 vlt. leſſe for ber. 180. 32 with for mith. 194. 16. ſinues for ſinners. 198. 21. for entreth ſeemeth. 204. 1 for which, vvith. 222. laſt. read foūd you pure and ſincere in his beloued Sonne. 241. 9 for dutie, dyet. 242. 21. for allovve, allure. 248. 3 for Ariſtophanes, Ariſtoxenes. 248. 14. put out the firſt vvith. 249. 15. for may, reade may ye. 251. 23. for ſoiled read ſailed. 254. 14. for to, a. 258. 1. for of, and. 258. 13. for iuice reade ſvveete. 258. 25.

Bei Fragen zur Produktsicherheit wenden Sie sich bitte an:
If you have any questions regarding product safety,
please contact:

Walter de Gruyter GmbH
Genthiner Straße 13
10785 Berlin
productsafety@degruyterbrill.com